M000288254

FIT TO SERVE

BECOMING WHAT YOU WERE CREATED TO BE

COACH POWERS

YWAM PUBLISHING
P.O. BOX 55787 SEATTLE, WA 98155

YWAM Publishing is the publishing ministry of Youth With A Mission. Youth With A Mission (YWAM) is an international missionary organization of Christians from many denominations dedicated to presenting Jesus Christ to this generation. To this end, YWAM has focused its efforts in three main areas: (1) training and equipping believers for their part in fulfilling the Great Commission (Matthew 28:19), (2) personal evangelism, and (3) mercy ministry (medical and relief work).

For a free catalog of books and materials, call (425) 771-1153 or (800) 922-2143. Visit us online at www.ywampublishing.com.

Fit to Serve: Becoming What You Were Created to Be

Published by YWAM Publishing
a ministry of Youth With A Mission
P.O. Box 55787, Seattle, WA 98155

13 12 11 10 09 1 2 3 4 5

ISBN 978-1-57658-517-7

Printed in the United States of America.

To my dad, Iron Mike Powers,
for sharing the passion of strength, power, and might

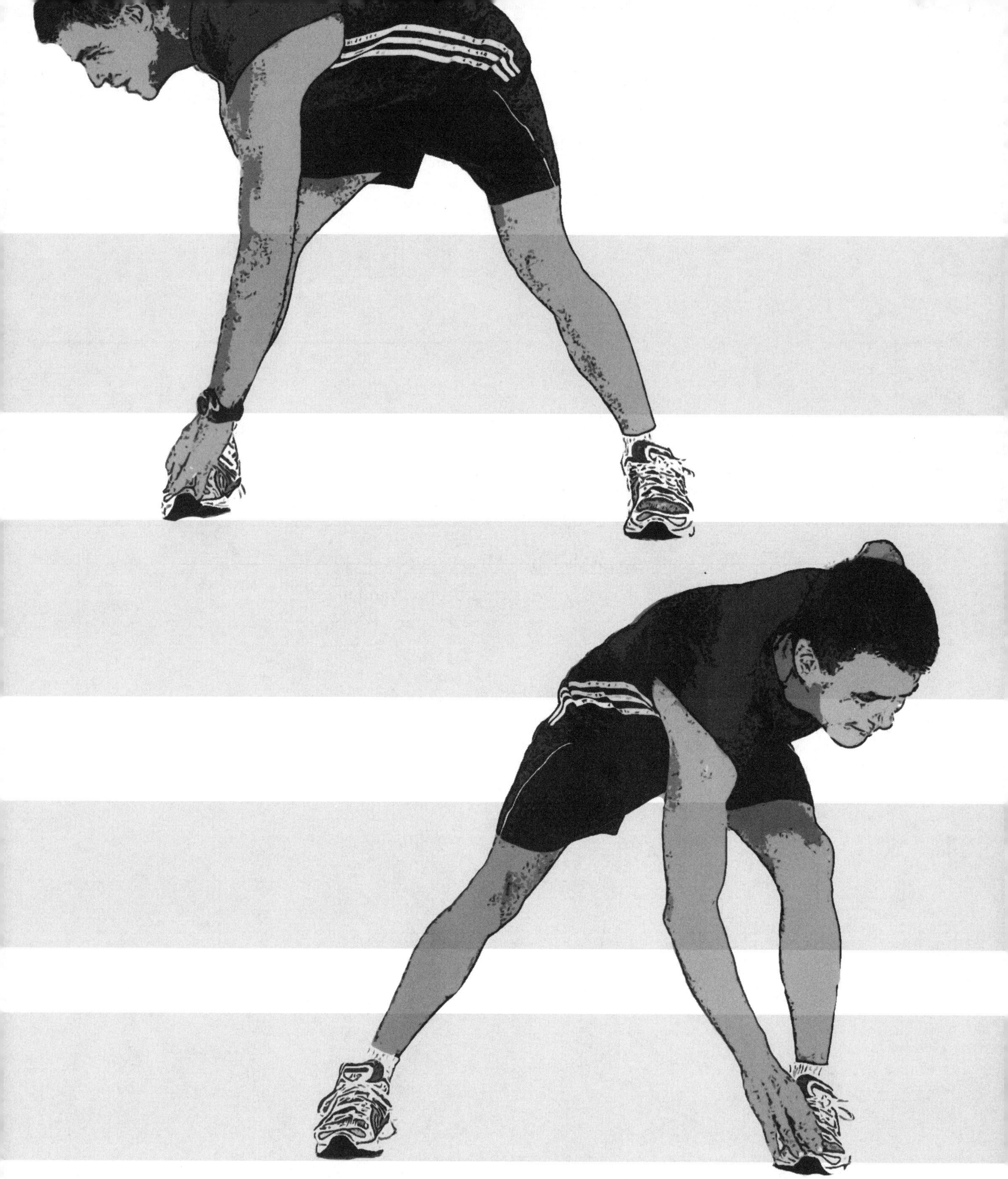

Fit to Serve is intended for informational and educational purposes only, and is not a substitute for medical advice. Please seek medical supervision before starting any exercise program or changing your diet. Neither the publisher or the author is engaged in rendering professional advice or services to the individual reader, and neither shall be liable or responsible for any loss or damage arising from any information or suggestion in this book.

foreword

Coach Tim Powers deserves the name "Coach." In a matter of five weeks, he proved to me that he could take someone who had just gone through surgery (a knee replacement and all the problems that follow) and prepare that person (me) to go to the Antarctic. The trip required physically demanding transfers from the ship to the rubber dingy, excursions across the water to get to shore, walks across ice and rocks among the penguins and sea lions, and entry into scientific stations in twelve locations. Before Coach Powers started working with me, I could never have made such an arduous journey.

Coach Powers has trained athletes from the National Football League and NASCAR as well as federal law enforcement and United States military professionals (including Navy Seals)—people who need to be fit to maintain a career on the cutting edge of their profession as well as people who are in life-and-death situations, where, if they are not fit, they will not survive. In Acts 1:1 Jesus first began to do, and then He taught. Coach Powers exemplifies this same model in that he lives and breathes fitness and therefore teaches it with great authority. In addition, through his winning personality and way of training, he makes you *want* to do better and become a more fit person.

As you work through this book or watch his routines on video or meet him and have him coach you in person—whichever way you engage with Coach Powers—you will be inspired by one of the best in the field to do better and become a stronger, fitter person. I happily commend Coach Powers to you as a person, as a coach, and as my friend.

Loren Cunningham
Founder of Youth With A Mission International
President of University of the Nations

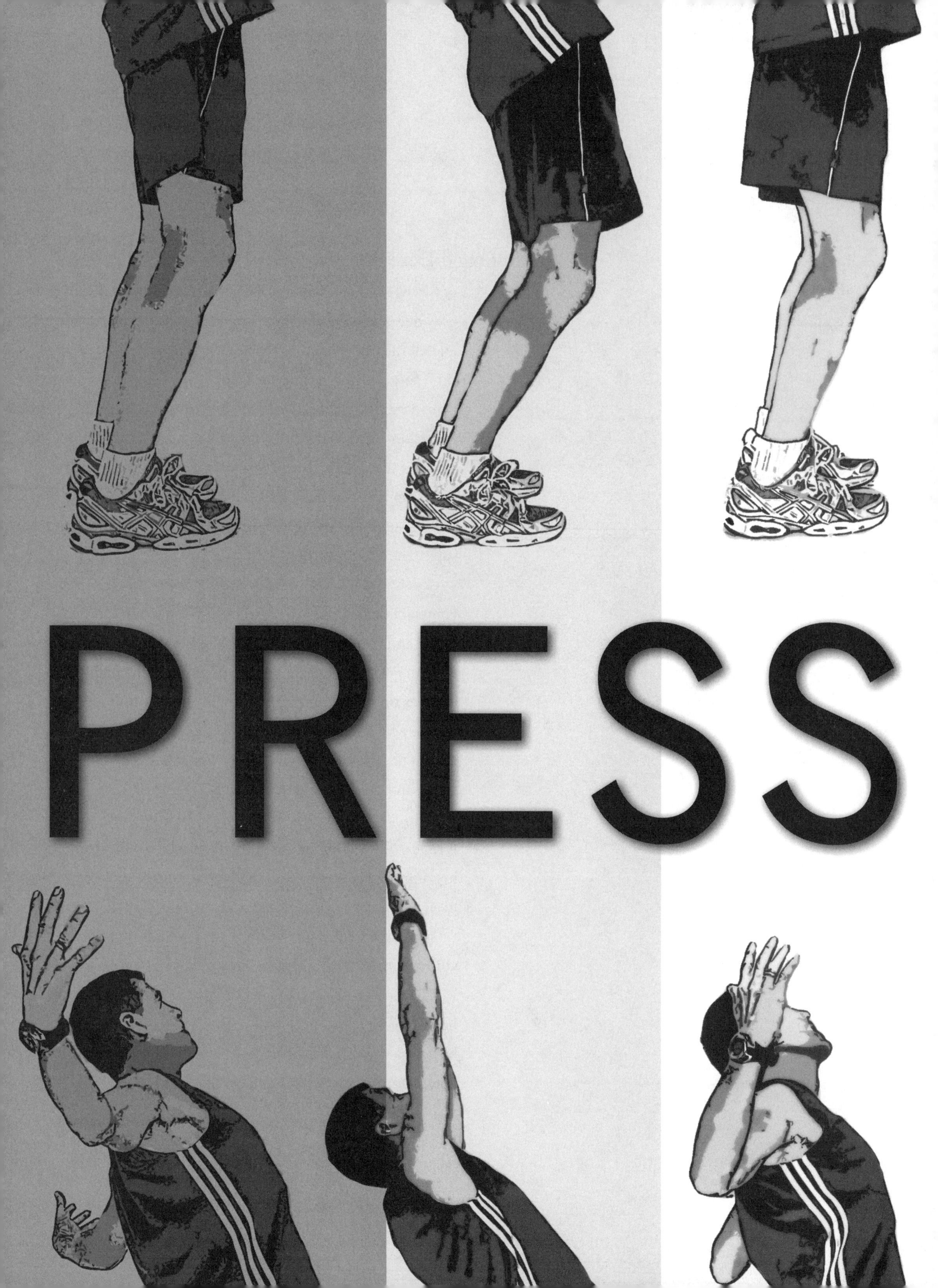
PRESS

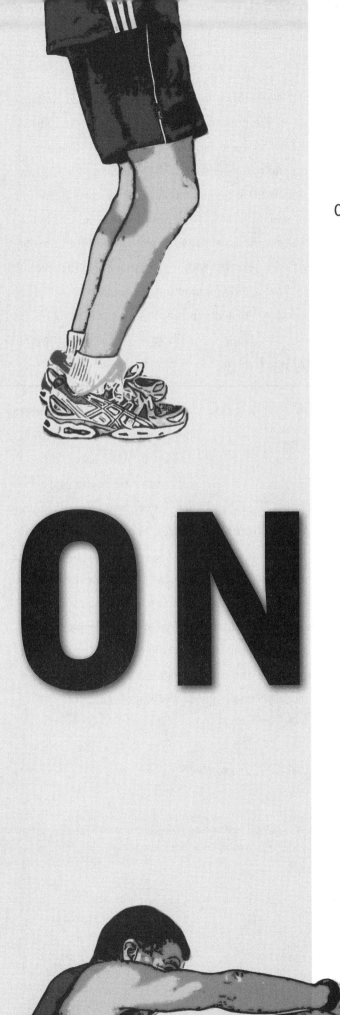

ON

introduction

Congratulations on picking up this book! You knew from the title alone that it was going to be a book about serving. Something in you knows that joy comes from helping others, that joy is found in giving, not in receiving. I'm sure you've heard this hundreds of times, but I think that you believe it.

May I ask you a personal question? Are you, right now, committed to doing everything you can to maximize your life? If you said yes, then this book was written for you. You're the type of person who is trying to become the best human being you can be.

Did you know that, in Hebrew, Adam means "human"? Yes, Adam of the Garden of Eden was the first human being. After Adam and Eve disobeyed God and ate the forbidden fruit, they fell from their position of being perfect, without defect. You and I are descendants of this fallen couple. To at least some degree, we battle this inheritance every day.

Even if inheriting fallen nature means that it will be an uphill struggle, I want to become what I was created to be. I want my life to have meaning. I want to carry out what God intended for my life before I was born. I want to wake up every morning excited about what the new day is going to bring, looking for adventure and fun. I want to have the energy and the vitality to see new places, meet new people, and experience new cultures. And I want to live a life of high quality for as long as I can. None of us knows with certainty what lies ahead, but, if possible, I choose quality versus quantity, hands down! Even though anything we will ever become occurs within the context of our relationships with other people, I don't want to be completely dependent on others as I live out the end of my life. My two grown daughters, Michelle and Krista, know to keep me out on

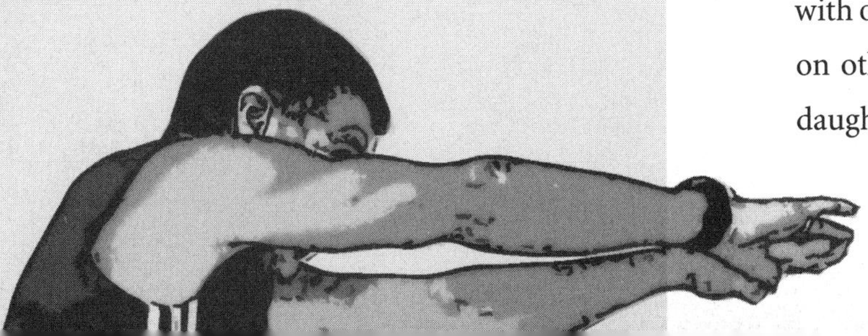

a grass soccer field when I'm nearing the end of my life so that, if possible, I can run my beloved sprints. They know that until it's time for the Lord to take me home, I want to be moving at full throttle. I hope to go back to my Creator at maximum intensity, shouting as loud as I can, "Here I come! I'm coming home, Father!"

How about you? What do you want for your life and the lives of your loved ones? You may say you want happiness, but what does it mean to be happy? Happiness is dependent on circumstances: You buy a new car and you're happy for a few days. You get a raise at work and it makes you happy for a while. Thinking about a vacation makes you feel happy until you actually go on that vacation. You constantly buy stuff and more stuff to keep yourself happy. You know what I'm getting at—happiness is temporary at best. We're happy for only fleeting moments.

"How about you? What do you want for your life and the lives of your loved ones?"

I don't want to be happy here and there, and now and then. No! I want to be fired up all the time! I want to be full of joy every day that I spend on this earth. You see, unlike happiness, joy is not dependent on circumstances. It's based on who we are and not on what we have. Joy is an attitude that comes from the deepest part of our being, and it's the greatest attitude we can have. Living an abundant life and prospering in all things means having radiant joy. It's our inheritance as Christians. I've written this book for believers. If you're a follower of Jesus, you're my target audience. Whether you're male or female, young or old, I've written this book for you.

I'm a fifty-four-year-old fitness guy. In 1957 my dad had me kneel down on the living room floor in our home in Green Bay, Wisconsin. It was after Thanksgiving, so of course it was freezing outside, fit for neither man nor beast. He knelt down beside me and proceeded to demonstrate to me how to do a classic pushup. After showing me how to do it, he told me to assume the starting position and to do as many pushups as I could before my arms buckled. He told me to do pushups every day for the rest of my life. And you know, I have—all of my life. I believe that the Lord spoke to my dad and told him to tell me that he wanted me to be involved in a lifetime of fitness. What I didn't know until recently was that the Lord wants me to tell you how and why to get as physically fit as possible for the rest of your life.

So yes, this is a fitness book, but not just another fitness book, sitting on a bookshelf. This is a book based on the idea that God is the one who wants us fit. The Bible is filled with encouragement for us to begin obeying him in this area. This is a book designed to motivate you to obedience. You can have the energy, the resolve, and the will to press on and finish the race in your life. You can run the race to fulfill the assignment God has given you to make this world a better place. Most important, I want to help you help others. I want them to see God in you and want what you have in life.

My mission is to help you become...

Fit to Serve!

Coach Powers

Part One: **God Designed Us to Be Fit**

It's so unbelievably cool that we were created to be whole and perfect and amazing in body, soul, and spirit—and to be so in a way that glorifies the One who created us to relate to him unlike any of the rest of his creation.

Humanity is the pinnacle of God's creative work, not only in our role as image-bearer, able to relate, to rule, and to represent God, but also as the crown jewel in being formed by God's hand (all the other creatures were spoken) and breathed into with God's breath, making our created bodies truly a masterpiece without equal.

Based upon this wholeness and integration, I offer this definition of physical fitness: Physical fitness is wholeness in the body and within one's spirit. It is the ability to perform vocational and recreational tasks without risk of injury and undue fatigue. It is wholeness in harmony and without defect.

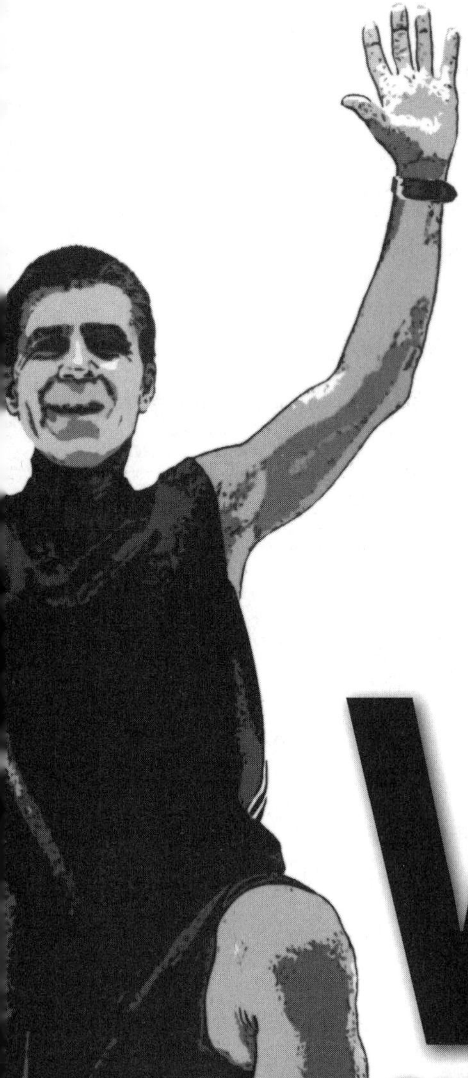

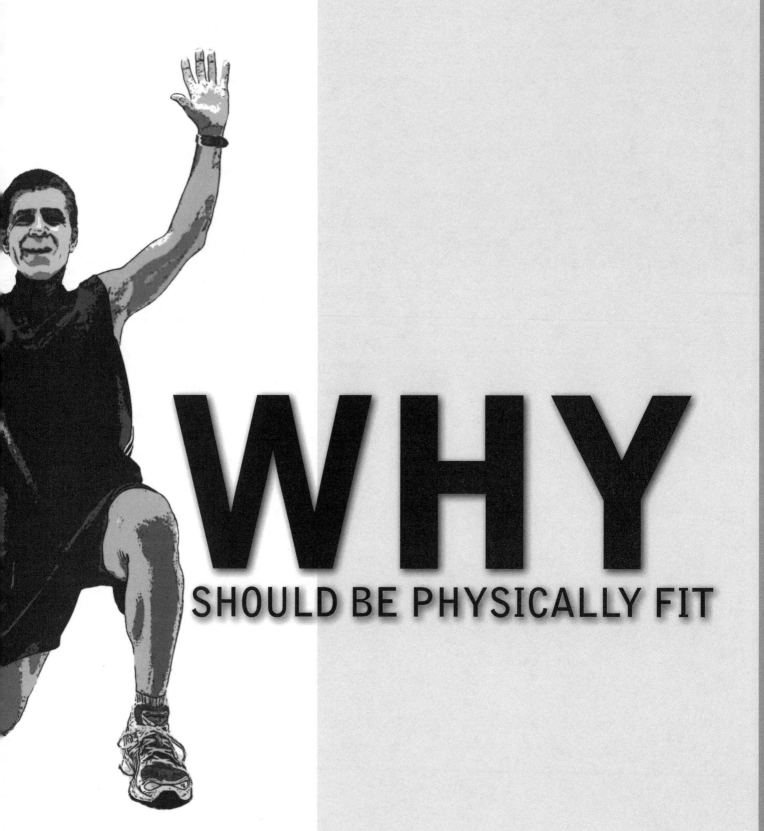

WHY
SHOULD BE PHYSICALLY FIT

WE

1

Many people I know, including non-Christians, think their bodies are inherently weak and undisciplined. Many Christians believe their flesh is not only weak but evil as well. The Bible refers to our flesh as the "old man" in us. The Bible tells us to crucify the flesh and nail it to the cross daily. But in this case it is talking about our sin nature, that part of our soul that was fallen and cursed to death before Jesus came, died on the cross, and redeemed us—spirit, soul, and body.

Remember, before Adam and Eve fell from their original position, their bodies were perfect and without defect. Our bodies had a divine nature, not the fleshly old man. Death, decay, and disease weren't part of the equation until after man sinned. Here's a question for you. Why did Jesus come to the earth and assume human form? Most Christians give answers like these:

1. He came to seek and save the lost.
2. He came to heal the sick and raise the dead.
3. He came to die for our sins.

These are all correct answers, but they aren't the only reason he came. In Isaiah 61:1, Isaiah says the Messiah would be anointed to bring good news to the poor, to comfort the brokenhearted, to proclaim the release of captives, to announce freedom for prisoners.

In a nutshell, Jesus came to set us free. When Jesus died on the cross, he accomplished that. He went down to hell, ripped the keys of sin and death out of Satan's hands, and redeemed us—spirit, soul, and body.

As of that moment in history, Satan and his minions no longer had power and authority over us. We were instantly redeemed. We are, right now, free to ascend to the heavenlies. The only power Satan has over us is when we give him power by sinning. If we don't sin, Satan has no power over us. It's that simple.

First, Be Fit Because Jesus Set Us Free

The first reason we should become physically fit is because Jesus paid for our freedom. He redeemed us completely. Calling for an appropriate response to this redemption, in Romans 12:1 (my paraphrase), the apostle Paul pleads with us to give our bodies to God because of all he has done for us. He asks us to let our bodies be a living and holy sacrifice—the kind God will find acceptable. This is truly the way to worship him.

Do you think the body of Christ, the people who call themselves the church, are giving their bodies to God? I imagine your answer is no. All you have to do is look around in the pews and aisles when you're at church. Obesity and the diseases that come with it are not only pandemic in our society but are also rampant in our churches.

Second, Be Fit to Be Salt and Light

The second reason why Christians should be physically fit is identified in Matthew 5:13–16. Jesus says:

> You are the salt of the earth, but what good is salt if it has lost its flavor? Can you make it useful again? It will be thrown out and trampled underfoot as worthless. You are the light of the world—like a city on a mountain, glowing in the night for all to see. Don't hide your light under a basket! Instead, put it on a stand and let it shine for all. In the same way, let your good deeds shine out for all to see, so that everyone will praise your heavenly Father.

Jesus calls us to be salt and light to the world. Our appearance, energy, and behavior should make people around us thirsty to know why we are the way we are. Our electricity and brightness should penetrate the darkness so that people everywhere will say, "I want to be like them and have what they have."

PHYSICAL FITNESS = FREEDOM TO REJOICE

Jesus gave us a new heart and set us free, free to be all we are meant to be. In 2 Timothy 1:7, we learn that God gave us a fearless spirit of power, love, and self-discipline. God gave us this fearless spirit to overcome the sinful desires of our "old man" flesh. We should get physically fit so that the world around us sees that we are "walking our talk." In 1 Corinthians 9:25–27, the apostle Paul spells out in no uncertain terms:

> All athletes practice strict self-control. They do it to win a prize that will fade away, but we do it for an eternal prize. So I run straight to the goal with purpose in every step. I am not like a boxer who misses his punches. I discipline my body like an athlete, training it to do what it should. Otherwise, I fear that, after preaching to others I myself might be disqualified.

The bottom line is that God wants the fallen world to see his son Jesus when they look at us, period!

Third, Be Fit to Honor Him

The third reason that God wants you to get physically fit is to honor him in reverence and awe. It doesn't get any more serious than when the apostle Paul exhorts us in 1 Corinthians 6:19–20:

> Don't you know that your body is the temple of the Holy Spirit, who lives in you and was given to you by God? You do not belong to yourself, for God bought you with a high price. So you must honor God with your body.

Taking care of the "temple" by keeping our bodies healthy and physically fit is one of the ways we can be obedient to this command to honor God with our bodies. And just like all the commands the Lord has given us, it's really for our own benefit. When we're obedient, we're the ones who get blessed. I believe that the Father God wants his children as physically fit as possible in these end days. He wants us to have the energy and vital force to accomplish his plans on earth.

Physical fitness should be a joyous thing. It's something you get to do, not something you have to do. I run twenty to forty 100-yard sprints every morning, six days a week. When I'm sprinting at my maximum capacity, I know that I'm the most alive I can ever be. When I'm sprinting, I'm utilizing all 650 muscles and 206 bones in my body at the same time. That feeling of my heart pounding through my chest and my lungs sucking air is like no other feeling I can describe. When I'm running sprints, I feel so very close to God. I believe that Jesus smiles when I sprint and the angels get excited. Sprints are "church" for me.

Being physically whole and unlimited in my movements is such a privilege. No one knows what the next day will bring, so make the most of the body that the Lord has given you right now. Don't wait until tomorrow or next week; start right now. Make a commitment in your soul right now. If you've been negligent or sinful in not giving your body to God, it's not too late. It's never too late. Ask the Lord to forgive you, and then be prepared to take that first great step of faith. If you step across the Physical Fitness Faith Line and show up, God will do the rest! If you do the possible, God will do the impossible. He will make your physical fitness grow and develop.

>> *tip:* Eat and Move

For the end of each chapter, I thought it would be fun to present you with some Eat and Move options while you are reading this book. We'll talk soon about thermogenesis (the process of creating heat and energy), but for now let's get you started on the path to physical fitness by eating and moving. It takes as little as forty-five seconds to increase your metabolic rate through a whole body movement. And if you choose a food snack that is loaded with energy, vitamins, and minerals, you'll ramp up your metabolic rate as well.

Here we go: There's nothing better than a glass of refreshing water. Grab your water bottle or an eight-ounce glass of the universal lubricant! Now take a deep breath and enjoy drinking exactly what your body needs.

WE ARE MADE IN GOD'S IMAGE

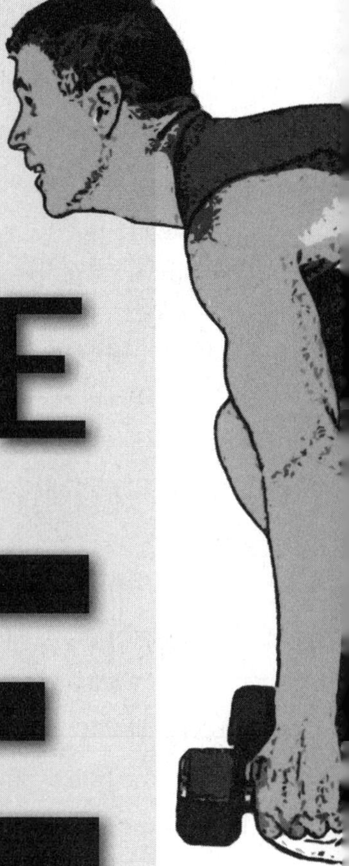

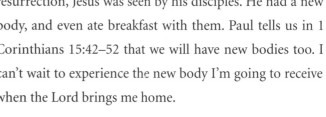

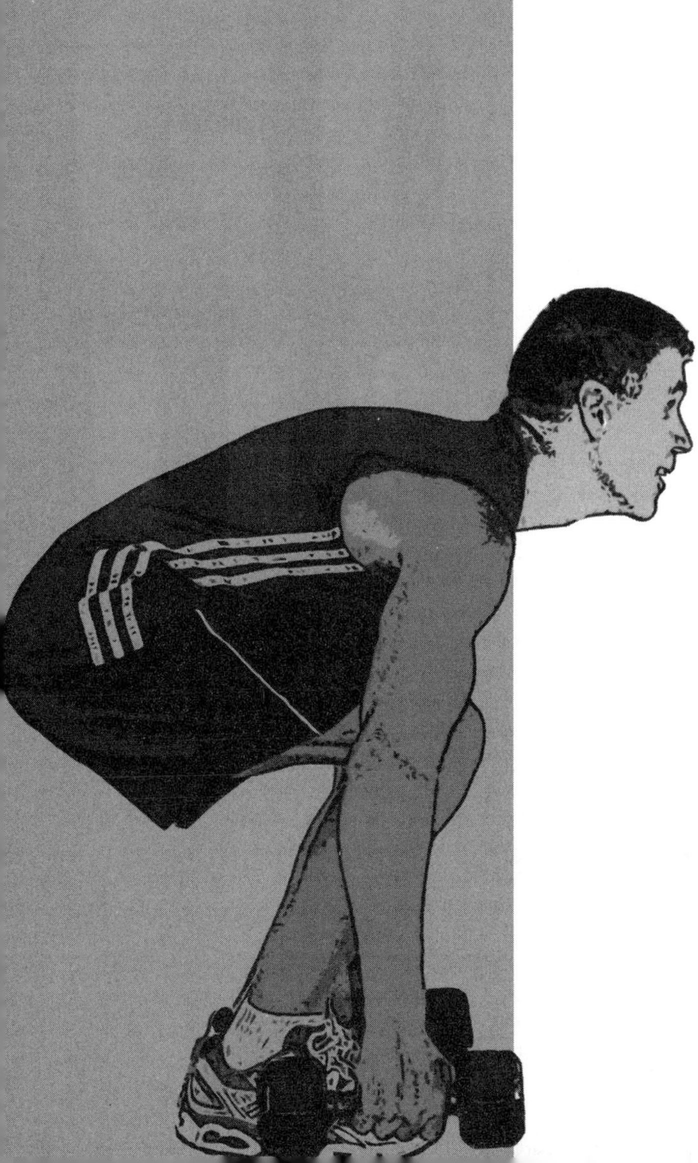

2

We all know the account of creation in the book of Genesis, chapters one and two. After God created human beings, the Bible says that he blessed them. That must have been a blessing with some serious power behind it, because right after the blessing he told them to be fruitful and multiply. He told them to fill the earth and govern it, to reign over the fish in the sea, the birds in the air, and all the animals that scurry along the ground.

Can you picture Adam calling for a male lion to come over to him so that he could pet him or maybe wrestle with him? Watch him as he rides atop a rhinoceros's bare back. See him punching an elephant's shoulder affectionately, and see the elephant wince from the pain of the punch.

I'm sure that both Adam and Eve had this level of physical prowess. They were physically perfect, strong, and intelligent. Their movements must have been graceful, fluid, and effortless. Sometimes we get rare glimpses of what we lost when they sinned against their own bodies by disobeying the Lord's command. You've probably heard about a grandma who reacts without thinking to the grandchild pinned under the frame of an automobile. In an enormous expression of love, she picks up the back of the vehicle, lifts the wheels off the ground, and frees her grandchild. How is that possible? Such examples demonstrate superhuman power. They remind us what we used to be before the Fall.

Our spirit and our mind tell us there is only so much we can restore to our bodies in a fallen world. We know that we will be completely restored in our next life. After the resurrection, Jesus was seen by his disciples. He had a new body, and even ate breakfast with them. Paul tells us in 1 Corinthians 15:42–52 that we will have new bodies too. I can't wait to experience the new body I'm going to receive when the Lord brings me home.

In the meantime, God wants to restore as much as possible so that we can accomplish our destiny and finish the race set before us. In Psalm 30:2, David called out to the Lord and God restored his vitality. As we cry out, we are doing our part. The Lord helps those who are already moving. Doing our part is simply showing up. This is an act of faith. God acts when we have faith. In fact, we can't please him unless we have faith (Hebrews 11:6).

When I was a brand-new baby Christian in 1980, Isaiah 40:31 was my favorite Scripture.

> Those who wait on the LORD will find new strength. They will fly high on wings like eagles. They will run and not grow weary. They will walk and not faint.

To "wait on" or trust in the Lord means to have a confident expectation. It means you believe without doubting. When you believe without doubting, you become totally immersed in that thing you are choosing to believe. You have a burning desire to believe. You want it fervently. This is the kind of trust you must have in order for your physical fitness to be restored to the highest degree. You'll have to pray to the Lord and be faithful and diligent day after day, week after week, month after month, and year after year.

From what I've read and what I've heard, the apostle John was a believer in physical fitness. He lived well into his nineties. In one of his letters to us, 3 John 2 (my paraphrase), he prays that we will prosper abundantly in all things, and that we will enjoy great health, as he knows that our souls are prospering. One evangelist says that we will never be more physically fit than our soul is.

So, to live the abundant life, full of maximum joy, we must seek fitness for our body and our soul; the two go hand in hand. If you are a Christian who is addicted to the Word, seeking to know God more every minute, then your soul is already fit. If your soul is fit but your body is not, all you have to do is step into obedience and be faithful with your body. If you do, I believe that you will be restored at a supernatural pace. That's what John was praying for in 3 John 2.

"God wants to restore as much as possible so that we can accomplish our destiny and finish the race set before us."

I've experienced this with wonderful, God-loving Christians that I've had the privilege of training. I worked with the founder of one of the largest missionary organizations in the world. He could only ascend and descend steps by painfully taking one at a time. He'd have to step up with his right foot and then bring his left foot up to the same step. Within two weeks of working with this man of great faith, he could go up and down steps in an unrestricted manner. Two weeks! How could someone make that kind of progress? You can experience this joy of fitness too. Simply show up, do your part, and act faithfully. God will do the rest.

>> *tip:* Eat and Move

Feeling hungry? Eat an apple, and make sure to taste how delicious it is. You'll be hard pressed to find anything that is more nutritious than this incredible fruit.

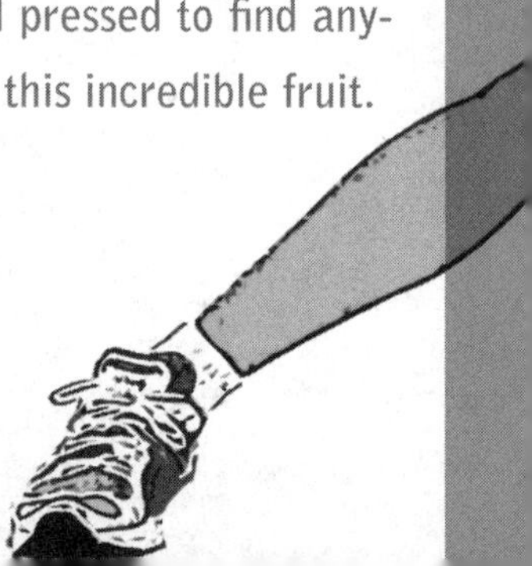

3

WE'RE FEARFULLY AND WONDERFULLY MADE

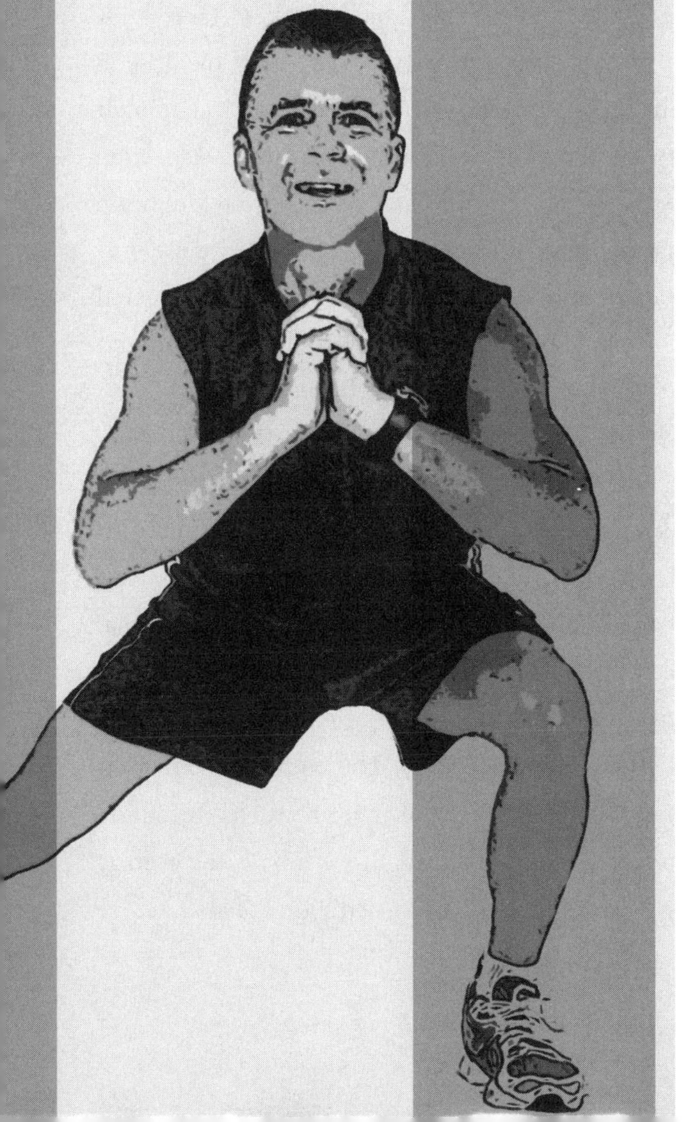

You probably have a favorite person from the Bible (other than Jesus, of course) that you would like to meet some day. My favorite is King David—I can't wait to meet him! Yes, King David was a ladies' man, but he was also a man's man. From the description in 1 Samuel 16:12, we see that he was dark and handsome, with beautiful eyes. In chapter seventeen of the same book, in verses 34–36, we also see that he was quick, agile, strong, and powerful. He took on bears and lions. He would catch them by their jaws and club them to death.

For ten years of my life, I had the awesome opportunity and responsibility of training military and police personnel in defensive tactics. One of the levels of force in which I instructed these soldiers and officers was the use of impact weapons, such as clubs and sticks. Over these years, I practiced hitting objects as hard and as fast as I could.

One time I was out on a fitness run when a big, yellow dog leapt at me. As it lunged for my throat, I side-stepped it and hit his head with a metal pipe as hard as I could. But my blow didn't slow him down. He kept coming after me. Fortunately, I was able to move out of his territory, and he dropped back. At the time of that assault, I had performed countless practice strikes. Yet my strike hadn't stopped that dog. That makes me realize how fit David was, to drop a lion and a bear! Imagine the level of force and intensity that David and his mighty men were capable of. Physically fit? I'd say they were—to the highest level attainable. David must have had a keen insight into the wonder of the human body. Aside from saying that we are fearfully and wonderfully made, take a look at what he says in Psalm 139:13–17:

> You made all of the delicate, inner parts of my body and knit me together in my mother's womb. Thank you for making me so wonderfully complex! Your workmanship is marvelous—and how well I know it. You watched me as I was being formed in utter seclusion, as I was woven together in the dark of the womb. You saw me before I was born. Every day of my life was recorded in your book. Every moment was laid out before a single day had passed. How precious are your thoughts about me, O God! They are innumerable! I can't even count them; they outnumber the grains of sand! And when I wake up in the morning, you are still with me!

The Lord God is talking about you and me here. Do you think the Lord loves David more than you? Not a chance! You are fearfully and wonderfully made. You are the apple of his eye.

Our bodies are important to God. They're important because, with them, we carry out our mission assignments to further the purposes of his kingdom. Our assignments are so crucial in the battle against the forces of darkness and evil that the Godhead must have invested a tremendous amount of time, thought, planning and energy into creating us. He composed us of seventy-five trillion cells and divided them into two hundred types. He designated every type to perform a particular job, whether absorbing nutrients from food, secreting hormones, detoxifying poisons, or the many other jobs necessary to maintain bodies.

From our smallest cell to the totality of our being, he organized us to do the work of living. It is not our structure that makes us what we are, but the way in which every part of us functions as a uniquely contributing part of the whole. Each one of our seventy-five trillion cells finds the meaning of its individual existence through participation in the miraculous project of us as human beings. And any one of these cells can be removed from our body and placed in a dish of nutrient broth, and it will go right on living and growing.

Many Christians define the soul as the mind, will, and emotions. At the very center of the soul lies the brain. The brain is the supreme survival organ created by God. I want to thank Dr. John J. Ratey for the helpful brain information in his book *A User's Guide to the Brain.* The following has been adapted from it.

There are a hundred billion neurons in the human brain, and roughly ten times as many other cells that have non-computational roles. Each of these hundred billion neurons have anywhere from 1 to 10,000 connections to other neurons. This means that the theoretical number of different patterns of connections possible in a single brain is approximately 40,000,000,000,000,000—forty quadrillion. Most astrophysicists calculate the volume of the known universe, in cubic meters, to be roughly ten to the eighty-seventh power. Our forty quadrillion potential interconnections and electrochemical configurations amount to a knee-bending and mind-staggering number—ten to the trillionth power. Therefore, even though modern-day scientists estimate that we use only 6 to 10 percent of our mental capacity, I believe that God has hard-wired our brains to know and understand him. Some day our true capacities will be realized.

How much do you think you're worth in monetary terms? Chemistry professors used to say that a person's market worth, from a strictly chemical standpoint, was about thirty-two dollars. But in recent years, this view has changed dramatically. Scientists now calculate that the electronic energy in the hydrogen atoms of your body is equivalent to a week's worth of electricity for a large, highly industrialized country. The atoms in your body contain a potential energy of more than eleven million kilowatt hours per pound. By this estimate, the average person is worth about eighty-five billion dollars.

The electrons in the atoms of your body are not just particles of matter; they are waves of living energy. And, in a way that I don't understand, scientists say these waves ripple out, spreading themselves in patterns of light, and as they move, they sing. Not only do they sing, they also shine. We're each a glistening, radiating, gleaming form.

Add to all this the fact that trying to reproduce your mind mechanically would cost billions of dollars. I pray that you're beginning to see yourself for what you really are: an amazing, infinitely valuable creature—God's masterpiece.*

>> *tip:* Eat and Move

Get energized by taking five deep breaths. Slowly begin to inhale through your nose and mouth, filling the lungs to maximum capacity. Then slowly exhale, gently pushing out every last bit of air. Repeat for all five breaths.

"I pray that you're beginning to see yourself for what you really are: an amazing, infinitely valuable creature—God's masterpiece."

The way that the human body is created from conception, and the way it can move under its own power is called vital force. This force is the life God breathed into us after molding us from clay. The more physically fit we are, the greater our vital force. I cry out to the Lord God by training and disciplining my body, and he restores my vital force. We're training our bodies to tune our spirits.

* Author adaptation taken from John J. Ratey, *A User's Guide to the Brain* (New York: Abacus, 2003), 9–11.

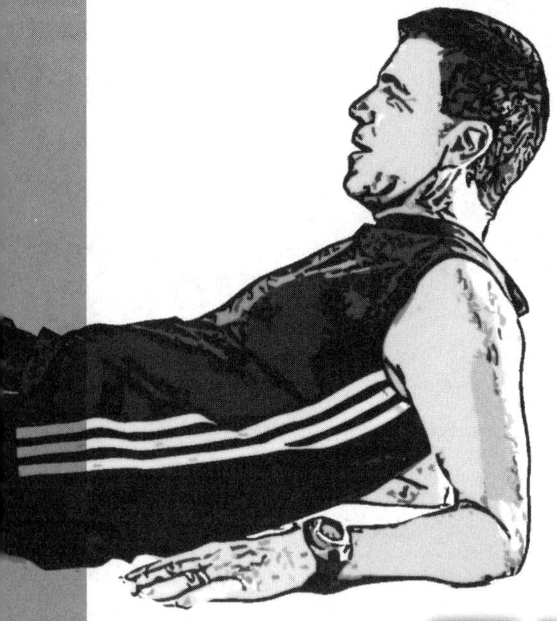

THE TEMPLE: HOW MADE

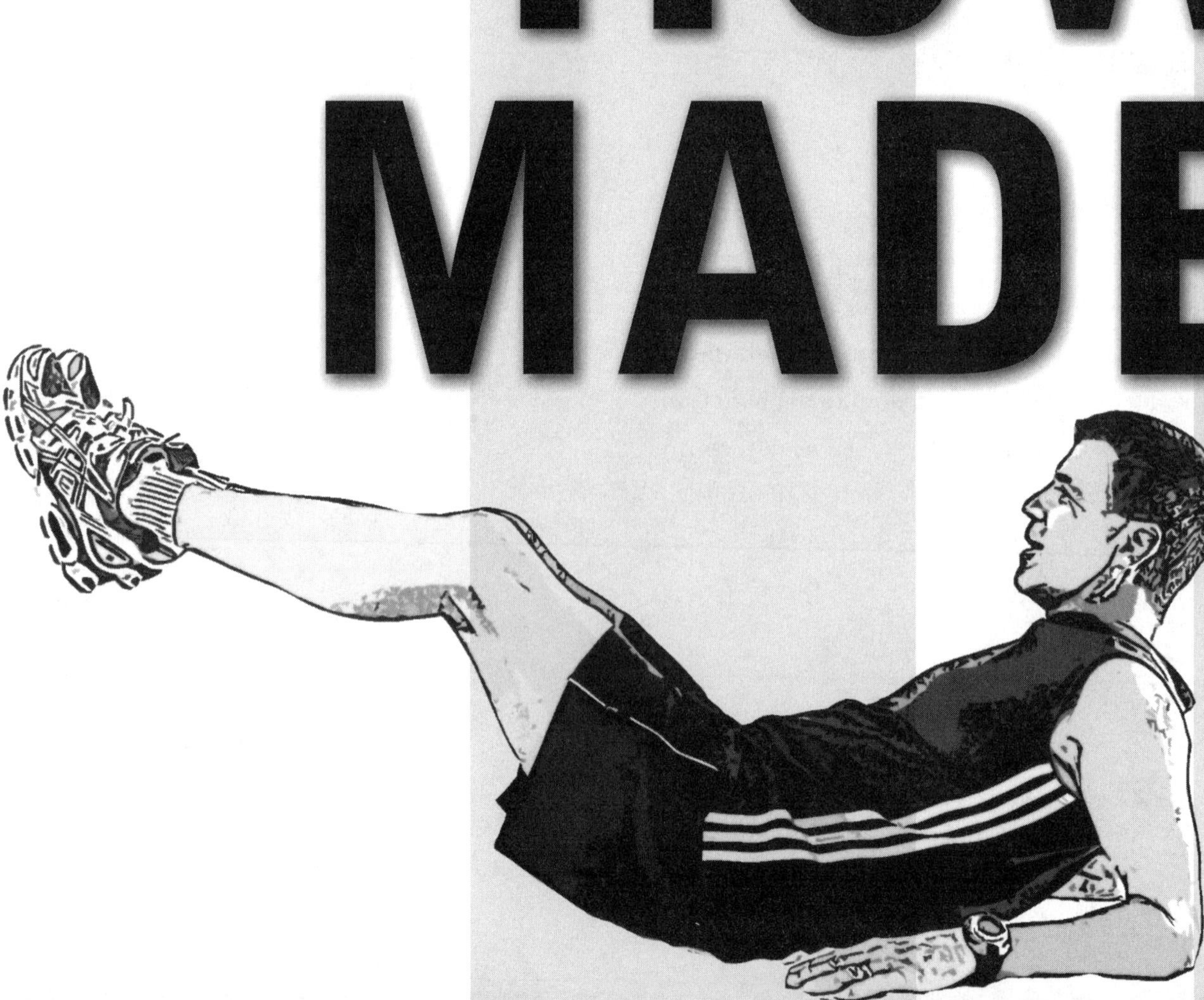

4

GOD US

In Alvin Toffler's book *The Third Wave,* he states that the highest form of power on earth is knowledge. I'm sure that you've heard the adage "Knowledge is power." Increasing your knowledge will provide you many advantages! But knowledge in and of itself doesn't do anything to improve your life or make this world a better place to live. Knowledge without action is stagnant and dead. Many have increased their knowledge but haven't applied their knowledge.

I realize that this will be the longest chapter so far, and maybe even a little slow reading. But I want to empower you and equip you with the basic understanding and tools that you will need to create your own unique physical fitness action plan, no matter where you are right now on planet Earth. It's very important for you not only to realize and perceive the marvel of your body but also to understand how it functions.

When I was in college studying for my undergraduate degree, I was required to take a class called Art Appreciation. Even though it was a required course, I loved it. I especially enjoyed studying the historical examples of architecture. The buildings and structures, and the periods in which they were constructed in human history, captured my imagination. I couldn't wait to get to class and see what I'd learn next. My favorite architecture was from the Greco-Roman period. From the Pantheon to the Colosseum to the Vatican—the buildings mesmerized me.

However, none of those magnificent structures can compare to the architectural design that the Lord used in creating our bodies. If we look at the human body as the temple of the Holy Spirit, the living, moving, modern-day ark of the covenant, it is absolutely the most incredible structure ever designed. It is a marvel of architecture, complete with domes (the skull), windows (the eyes), arches (the ribs), columns (the leg bones), and thousands of miles of passageways (the blood vessels).

The human body is a temple blazing with activity. It is always building, renovating, reproducing, and growing. It converts energy from one form to another, it sends and receives messages, it fends off intruders, and it performs extraordinary balancing acts. God made our bodies to function in a whole brain–whole body, integrated manner. We function chemically, electrically, and mechanically. The chemicals in our bodies are processed to release their energy in the form of high-energy electrons, the same sort of energy as electricity.

Adenosine triphosphate, or ATP, is the universal power source for all seventy-five trillion of your cells. Its energy is what drives your molecular motors. It activates muscles and gives nerve cells the power to make electricity to transmit signals from the brain to the body and from the body back to the brain. If you want more electricity, you have to produce it. You produce it by developing your physical fitness and vital force. The only way you're going to increase your vital force is by crying out to the Lord and asking for it through a burning desire and focused prayer, along with getting yourself moving.

The human body has ten integrated systems, each with its own job, but all highly interdependent. I want to acknowledge and thank the National Geographic Society for its exhaustive work in *Incredible Voyage: Exploring the Human Body.* This next section on systems has been largely adapted from their work.*

The Skeletal System

Your body contains 206 bones. Bones are the anchors to which the muscles attach. They act as levers and hinges for your daily activities; they are strong and sturdy, yet lightweight. They also cradle and protect your vulnerable organs. They house the cellular factories that produce your blood. And they act as storehouses for phosphorus and calcium. Bones make up 20 percent of your body's total mass.

The Muscular System

There are more than 650 muscles in your body, and they account for more than half of your body mass. Muscles provide the force for every one of your movements. They help you run, speak, sing, play music, and create art. There are three types of muscles: smooth, cardiac, and skeletal.

Smooth muscles are involuntary muscles, because they contract without conscious thought. For example, smooth muscles line the walls of your blood vessels and internal organs, helping move blood through the arteries and propel food through your stomach and intestines.

Cardiac muscle, found only in the heart, pushes blood out of your heart and throughout your body. Developing your physical fitness will strengthen both pump portions of your heart: the powerful left ventricle which sends the blood out into your body, and the right ventricle which sends blood back to your lungs to be reoxygenated. Your heart will contract an amazing two-and-a-half billion times in your lifetime.

Skeletal muscle attaches to your bones. These muscles control movements that are voluntary, that is, subject to your conscious choice. You choose to smile, run, jump, exercise, or sing a song.

Your muscles and skeleton move according to the lever principle. In this way the Lord made us to be very machine-like. When we move our bodies, bones serve as levers and joints act as hinges. Skeletal muscles supply the force. So by increasing the strength of your muscles

* *Incredible Voyage: Exploring the Human Body* (Washington, D.C.: National Geographic Society, 1998), 67–114.

you increase the available force to move your body with greater ease. By the way, it takes sixteen muscles to frown and only eight to smile. Not only is smiling more economical, but it brings you and others joy and peace.

The Circulatory System

As one poet said, blood is the color of life. It transports oxygen, nutrients, enzymes, proteins, and hormones to nourish all seventy-five trillion cells in your body. Your blood makes up about 8 percent of your body weight. Your heart drives the blood throughout your body, and arteries carry oxygenated blood to the large regions of your brain, torso, arms, and legs. Smaller vessels called capillaries transfer blood to each individual cell. Strenuous exercise increases the number of these capillaries, thus delivering more of everything good throughout your body. The pulmonary artery transports the deoxygenated blood back to the heart where it is pumped to the lungs to be reoxygenated, and also helps carry cellular waste out of the body.

In the time it took you to read this sentence, over three million of your red blood cells died. Fortunately, the Lord created red bone marrow in your body to replace the cells. And, should your kidneys detect that the red blood cells are not providing you with enough oxygen, they will order the marrow to produce even more.

Incidentally, the average adult carries approximately ten to thirteen pints of blood. But people who exercise regularly produce and carry fourteen to sixteen pints of blood. More blood permits a higher level of functioning and allows a better quality of life.

The Respiratory System

Your respiratory system includes the lungs and connecting tubes, which bring oxygen into the body and get carbon dioxide out. Without a fresh supply of oxygen you would die within minutes. When you exercise, you breathe rapidly because your muscles are using more oxygen. The respiratory system starts processing air as soon as you inhale it through your mouth and nose. The nasal passages immediately filter, warm, and humidify the air.

Breathing is automatic. While you can regulate the rate and depth of your breathing to some extent, it is mostly run from the brain's involuntary centers. When you inhale, the diaphragm—a sheet of muscle that forms the floor of the chest cavity—contracts, pulling downward to enlarge that cavity. This creates a lower air pressure in your lungs than exists outside the body, so air flows into the lungs. When you exhale, you reverse this process. The diaphragm muscle relaxes, the chest cavity shrinks, and pressure within the lungs builds. This causes a pressure differential in the other direction, and air gushes out. Just consider the creativity and fun the Lord must have had when he designed you. Each one of your lungs holds only a gallon or two of air, yet its internal surface area is as big as a tennis court. Imagine that!

"It takes sixteen muscles to frown and only eight to smile."

The Digestive System

The digestive system is like the respiratory system in that it works to provide your cells with the nourishment they need. The supplies come from what we eat and drink. This system is its own miracle as it transforms what we eat into energy. Even though Jesus told Satan that "people do not live by bread alone," we still need good food. Eating delicious food is one of the true pleasures of life. The Lord wants us to enjoy nutritionally dense, wholesome foods.

Foods, all foods, contain chemicals your body uses to live and thrive. If you don't get the nutrients that you need—the fatty acids, amino acids that make up proteins, carbohydrates, vitamins, and minerals—you can get sick and die. Remember our working definition of physical fitness. It is wholeness in the body and within one's spirit. It is the ability to perform vocational and recreational tasks without risk of injury and undue fatigue. It is wholeness in harmony and without defect. The food you eat is fuel for the repair and growth of your body, and the energy to carry out your assignment from the Lord.

Digestion begins in your mouth, where your teeth grind and mash food into smaller pieces. Three pairs of salivary glands secrete a mixture of mucous, water, and a digestive enzyme that immediately starts breaking down the food. Swallowing begins as a voluntary process, but then the involuntary pharynx muscle contracts, pushing the mashed up food to the esophagus, a muscular ten-inch tube leading to the stomach. The stomach, which is shaped like a fat letter *J*, does some mechanical processing of its own as the smooth muscles "roll" the contents around, and some chemical processing by producing gastric juice, a corrosive hydrochloric acid that kills microbes and begins to break down proteins.

"Physical fitness is wholeness in the body and within one's spirit."

About four hours after eating, your food passes into the small intestine, where the real digestion takes place. Most of the nutrients your body needs are extracted in the small intestine. Only an inch in diameter, the small intestine takes up most of the lower abdominal cavity. It measures about twenty feet in length, all coiled in place like sausage and held to the back of the abdominal wall by a thin sheet of connective tissue.

Once the small intestine completes its work, about three to ten hours after eating, the remaining material moves into the large intestine, or colon. The colon is about five feet long and three inches in diameter. It's coiled atop and around the small intestine. The colon reabsorbs water from all the spent digestive juices and returns it to circulation. (Aren't you just amazing?) With every bit of useful material now absorbed, what's left passes into the rectum and the anal canal for excretion.

The Urinary System

Your urinary tract removes liquid waste and regulates your body fluids. The key organs of this system are your kidneys. These two reddish-brown, bean-shaped organs sit in the back of your abdominal cavity. They filter and condition the blood, eliminate waste materials, balance the salts and liquidity of your bodily fluids, and keep your acid level just right.

The human body is mostly water—about 70 percent. Water is stored mainly in blood, muscles, and skin. Moving through your body, water distributes nutrients and chemicals, helps balance body temperature, dilutes toxins, and is the universal lubricant in which the complex chemical reactions of your metabolism occur. You can live without food for quite a while, but go without water for even a day and bad things happen.

In the end, your urinary system regulates the amount of water in your body, processing what you take in and getting rid of what you don't need. Water that is excreted is called urine. The composition and volume of your urine depends on what is happening throughout your body. If the body is in need of additional water, the kidneys will produce concentrated urine until you answer your thirst response. Similarly, when you exercise, your urine volume lowers, becoming more concentrated because your active body needs more fluid. Generally, the more yellow your urine, the more water you need.

The Skin System

As you have seen, your body is an amazing package, and that package is encased in a spectacular wrapping—skin. Your skin is your largest organ. It helps regulate body temperature, and protects against excess moisture and salt. It is full of sensors, or nerve endings, that measure temperature and, best of all, give you your sense of touch. It is also your main shield against infection from bacteria and viruses.

Your skin has an outer layer, the epidermis. It is constantly shedding and replacing cells. It serves as your body's armor. Underneath the epidermal skin layer is the dermis. This innermost dermis consists of tissue penetrated by blood and lymph vessels, nerves, hair, and sweat and sebaceous glands. At its base, the dermis connects to the underlying tissues. Because the skin is a visible organ, it sometimes acts as a barometer of your mood. It may turn red when you're embarrassed or angry, or white when you're frightened. The skin also provides an indication of your general health. How many times have you noticed the quality of someone's skin? Beautiful skin looks vibrant and healthy.

Even though your skin serves as your armor and protection, it is vulnerable. It's porous. Anything applied to your skin may penetrate to your underlying tissues. So a good rule of thumb is not to put anything on your skin that you can't eat (this includes tattoos as well as some sunscreens and deodorants).

The Nervous System

Up to this point I've shared what organs you have and how each functions within its system. However, all of your systems were created to work together. The master system that integrates all of the other systems is the nervous system. Its main function is communication. It receives and stores information about your inner and outer worlds. It initiates activity and carries electricity throughout your body.

Your nervous system never sleeps. It is constantly gathering data, shuttling this information to the brain for analysis, and then sending it down through the spinal cord to invoke action when necessary. The action of your nervous system keeps you alive, and when it shuts down, you are dead and going home to be with the Lord.

The Lord created and organized your nervous system brilliantly. The brain and spinal cord make up the central nervous system. Nerves branch out from the central nervous system, interlacing the tissues and bones of your body. These nerves are considered the peripheral nervous system. The basic unit of this system is the neuron, a cell that is capable of taking in information from all over your body and delivering the appropriate response.

Within the peripheral system are two subsystems: the somatic or voluntary system, and the autonomic. The somatic system is concerned with the nerves that register incoming stimulation and the body's voluntary responses. The somatic system performs conscious actions. The autonomic system takes care of involuntary processes, such as your heartbeat and breathing. This system operates on autopilot, running quietly in the background, but revving up instantly to respond to any challenge. It has the capacity to cause over 144 brain-to-body reactions in one to three seconds. Your glands charge your muscles for action, and your lungs fill rapidly with oxygen to fuel for flight or fight. The pupils of your eyes dilate to increase the acuteness of images you see. And some say this all happened as an evolution of your species. Not a chance in forty quadrillion!

The autonomic system is further divided into the sympathetic and the parasympathetic systems, which control internal organ reflexes. The sympathetic system responds to stress or emergencies. The parasympathetic system helps restore your body's resources, generally working to calm your body down.

And, finally, the nervous system sorts its tasks into sending or receiving. The sensory system transmits information from both the outside world and from within the body itself. Impulses travel from a sensory nerve to the central nervous system. The motor system is mostly voluntary. It sends impulses from the brain and spinal cord to your muscles and glands. When you decide to sprint or eat, impulses travel from motor nerves in the brain through the spinal cord and to the appropriate muscles.

The Endocrine System

Most of the chemical controls that keep you healthy and fit are invoked by powerful chemicals called hormones. These hormones are produced in endocrine glands. These glands are ductless—they simply release their hormones. Then these hormones are swept up by the bloodstream and taken to where their messages are read. Endocrine glands include the pituitary, adrenal, thyroid, parathyroid, pineal, thymus, pancreas, and the male and female sex glands, the testes and ovaries, respectively.

Hormones circulate through the body until they find the organs they are to influence. Almost every cell in your body is the target of at least one hormone. Each hormone works only on cells it recognizes. All of your seventy-five trillion cells have specific recognition sites for these hormones. These sites are called receptors.

Let's look briefly at an incredible physiological phenomenon called circadian rhythm. Scientists on the cutting edge of exercise science have discovered that each unique twenty-four hour cycle influences aspects of your body's function, including body temperature, hormone levels, heart rate, blood pressure, even pain threshold. Most of the hormones, chemicals, and neurotransmitters that build you up through repair and growth are produced between 3:00 and 6:00 AM. Your blood levels for these components will stay relatively high until noon. To take advantage of them, the best time to train or add muscle is in the morning, before you begin your morning duties and activities. There is a secondary production of these components between 3:00 and 6:00 PM, so the next best time to exercise is between these hours. Of course, the best time for you to exercise is when you can. I'll talk more about your exercise times in Part Two of this book.

"The best time for you to exercise is when you can."

The Reproductive System

I'll never forget when my thirteen-year-old nephew Jason was lamenting how his classmates were talking about girls. Apparently, they were making some sexually lewd comments. Jason said, "Hey! Keep your eyes on the Creator and off the creation. It's the reproductive system, not the recreation system."

I was so proud of Jason for his response. It takes maturity to understand the sacredness of a man and woman's sexual relationship. Sexual intimacy is to be an expression of God's love in marriage between a husband and a wife.

Human reproduction may not be quite the mystery that it once was, but it still remains a miracle. Think about it—one human growing inside of another! The human reproductive system is, like all of the systems in the body, chemical, electrical, and mechanical.

You may not realize it, but physically you are a product of your great, great grandparents. They have handed down physical, psychological, and emotional traits to you. Your ability to learn and perform various mental and physical tasks is 30 to 90 percent determined by your genetic heritage. A major league baseball pitcher who can hurl a fastball at ninety-seven miles per hour is born with that ability. However, in terms of your physical fitness development, you can make monumental improvements, no matter your genetic endowment.

In the next chapter, we'll see the benefits and blessings we receive when we give our bodies to God as a holy and living sacrifice.

>> *tip:* Eat and Move

Looking for protein density? Eat a small handful of raw almonds. Take your time in chewing (and enjoying) the nuts to ensure nutrient absorption and better digestion.

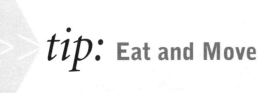

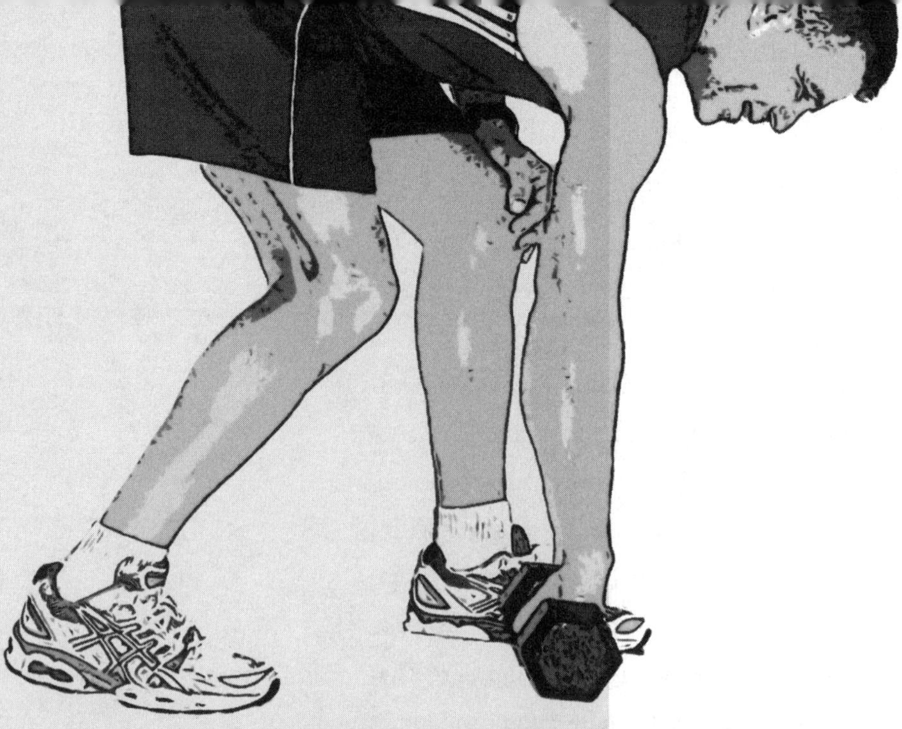

THE BENEFITS AND BLESSINGS

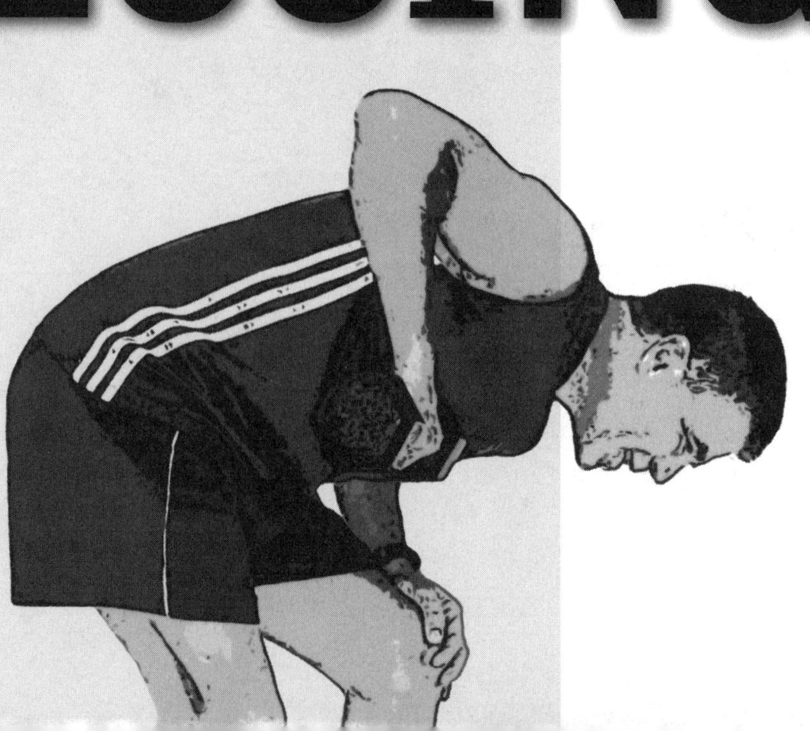

5

In the last chapter, I felt the need to establish the marvel of God's creation of your body. I did this so that you would be awestruck. But I also did it so you would be extremely grateful and have great respect for what God has done in you.

In earlier chapters, we've seen how the Word tells us to give our bodies to God, and that we are to discipline our bodies like athletes so that others will see for themselves that we are walking our talk. In Matthew 6:33, Jesus told us to first seek God's kingdom and his righteousness, and then all other things would be given to us. In other words, it's all about our motives—and God knows all of them. So, if your motives are to get as physically fit as possible for the glory and honor of God as expressed through your life, then the following are just some of the other things you can expect to receive.

The Benefits

Improving your level of physical fitness can benefit you in three primary ways: performing better, feeling better, and looking better.

Performing Better

Improving physical fitness allows the brain to think more creatively, to be sharp, focused, and articulate. Because your brain is an organic structure, it will function better with the additional blood, oxygen, and nutrients that you're sending it. Your brain will be able to send and receive information more efficiently to and from your body.

Physical fitness also improves the body's performance. Daily life is easier and injuries less likely (due to bending more before breaking) for those who are fit.

- Your strength, stamina, power, flexibility, coordination, and balance will improve as you become more physically fit.
- You'll have greater economy of motion.
- You'll have plenty of energy, and at the end of your day you'll sleep like a baby.
- You'll have greater body elasticity, a much larger range of motion in your joints, and what scientists call "amplitude"—the entire sweeping range of movement.
- If you do become injured, you'll heal much faster. In fact, if you have minor aches and pains, or a cold or flu, you'll find that movement helps speed your recovery.

Just writing about these benefits makes me want to get out and exercise. In fact, I'm going to take a break in my writing and go out for a power prayer walk. I'll be back to talk to you in a while.

Feeling Better

Did you ever notice that when you feel sick you're not as friendly and as loving toward people, especially your family? As your level of physical fitness spirals downward through poor choices, the quality and joy in your life bottoms out. In the opposite way, as your physical fitness increases, the quality of your life and your personal joy will rise.

- Your heart will function better because it's stronger and has more blood and oxygen.
- You'll breathe better because your lungs will be stronger and able to consume more oxygen.
- You'll be able to eat good food with greater digestion and less indigestion and constipation.
- You'll have better hearing, smell, taste, vision, and touch because the entire sensory apparatus is enhanced as your physical fitness improves.

Looking Better

How you look to yourself and others is also important. How you look speaks of your desire, discipline, and will.

- If you're lean and muscular, it says that you're eating right and exercising regularly.
- If your face and skin look radiant and young, it says that you're drinking the right amount of clean water and that you have a productive attitude and minimize the amount of stress in your life.
- If you move and look like a much younger person, it says that you must be staying flexible, mobile, and supple. It says that you must have a playful attitude and outlook in your life.
- If your body is lean and toned, you'll look great in your clothes. You'll be good-looking and attractive. People will be intrigued by why you are the way you are.

As you increase your degree of physical fitness, you can expect your self-esteem to rise accordingly. Often, as you get more physically fit, you're more comfortable with yourself. This allows you to be more friendly and loving toward others. Stressful things will become less stressful and more unimportant. You'll be more tolerant. People may even ask if you're taking "happy pills" or something. In all my years of personal training and presenting physical fitness seminars, I've met many godly people. They usually ask me how to improve their appearance. It's okay. God wants you to look your best.

The truth of the matter is that the spiritual laws of the universe express themselves in the physical laws. Consider the spiritual law of sowing and reaping. The Bible says that you will reap what you sow. If you want to increase your finances, help others financially. If you need help on a project, help someone on his project. If you're lonely and want companionship, reach out to others. This is a very simple concept to grasp, and it never fails. If you want to improve your physical fitness, you have to start being faithful and do your part. If you are faithful and act in obedience to God's Word, the spiritual blessings will overtake you.

The Blessings of Obedience

"Wherever you go and whatever you do, you will be blessed."
—Deuteronomy 28:6

This verse alone says it all. Wherever you go and whatever you do, you are blessed. I don't think I need any other motive to be obedient than this. How about you?

"The law of the LORD is perfect, reviving the soul."
—Psalm 19:7

Remember, the soul is defined as your mind, your will, and your emotions. When you're obedient to the Word, your mental faculties are revived.

"O LORD my God, I cried to you for help, and you restored my health."
—Psalm 30:2

When you read this verse, think "vital force." I don't know about you, but I want more vital force. When you show up for a workout, you are taking action. It is a form of "crying out" to the Lord for help. He will then restore your vitality.

"But you have made me as strong as a wild bull.... The godly will flourish like palm trees and grow strong like the cedars of Lebanon. For they are transplanted to the LORD's own house. They flourish in the courts of our God. Even in old age, they will still produce fruit; they will remain vital and green."
—Psalm 92:10, 12–14

So, the godly will be incredibly strong and will flourish. We'll remain vital and "green." To me, this sounds like the best anti-aging strategy I've ever heard or read about.

"Don't be impressed with your own wisdom. Instead, fear the LORD and turn your back on evil. Then you will have healing for your body and strength for your bones."
—Proverbs 3:7–8

If you and I are obedient to God's Word, our bodies will be healed, our bones will be strong.

My inspiration for writing this book was the desire to give you the motives and understanding of physical fitness so that you can carry out God's intended purposes for your life. No better scripture can justify your commitment to physical fitness than this one:

"Those who wait on the LORD will find new strength. They will fly high on wings like eagles. They will run and not grow weary. They will walk and not faint."
—Isaiah 40:31

I've shared most of these scriptures with my Christian friends. Many of them, maybe most of them, have responded by saying that it never occurred to them that these words were meant to be taken literally. They thought that these blessings were meant to be taken in a spiritual sense only and not in a bodily or physical sense. But I believe that God's Word means what it says literally. If you want to be blessed by God and physically fit, trust God and obey his Word.

>> *tip:* Eat and Move

How about a set of thirty jumping jacks? You can't perform these without getting a smile on our face, because they're so fun. Form an athletic stance and with your arms at your side, jump up and bring your hands together over your head while extending your feet six inches out to your sides. This exercise definitely adds some bounce to your steps.

Part Two: **Success Factors**

In John 1:1–5, it is written:

> In the beginning the Word already existed. He was with God, and he was God. He was in the beginning with God. He created everything there is. Nothing exists that he didn't make. Life itself was in him, and this life gives light to everyone. The light shines through the darkness, and the darkness can never extinguish it.

Jesus is a living force. So get addicted to Jesus, because he is life itself, both in the natural and in the spiritual. If you're going to stay the course in developing physical fitness for the rest of your life, you're going to need the spiritual power that only Jesus can give you. As one way of relating to Jesus, read the Bible every day and meditate on what it is telling you to do. Get addicted to the Word.

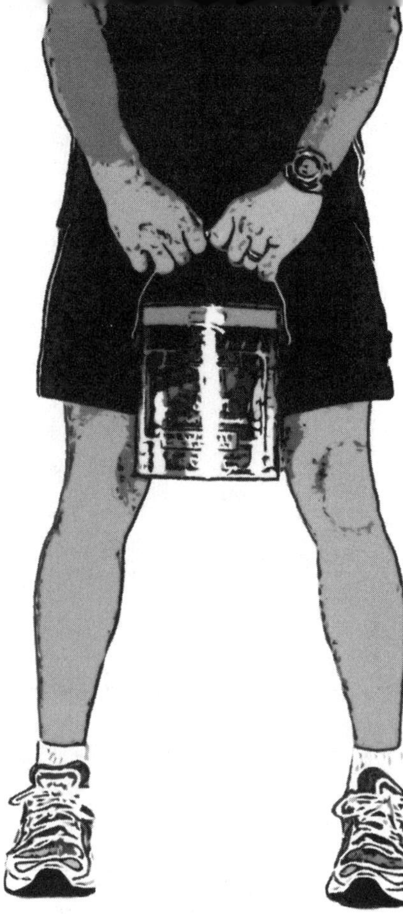

TIMELINE TO FITNESS

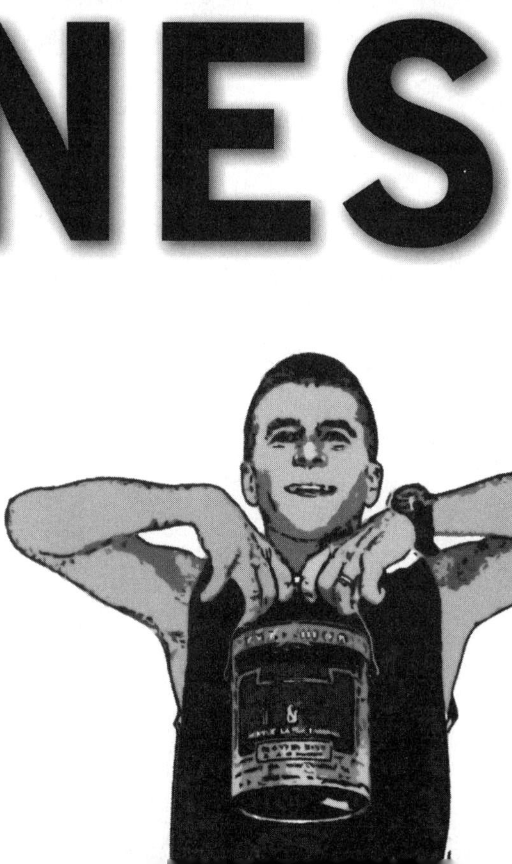

6

By all means, set yourself up for physical fitness success with a targeted timeline and the best information for healthy metabolism, nutrition, and sleep. Here are seven success factors to get you started.

Success Factor #1: Be Consistent—Show Up!

I've often jokingly stated in the seminars that I've presented over the past twenty-six years, that if I ever wrote a book on fitness, the words of the first chapter would read, "Be consistent. Be consistent. Be consistent. Be consistent. Be consistent. Be consistent. Be consistent. Be consistent...." Consistency is a critically important success factor in physical fitness because the body adapts over time to the traces left over from your previous workout. Dr. Ellington Darden, an exercise physiologist with Nautilus Fitness Equipment, says, if you don't exercise within four days of your last round of exercise, your body will reverse the training effect and you will begin to decondition. So you must decide to exercise on a regular basis. If you exercise now and then, all you're doing is keeping your body in a state of structural breakdown and potential injury. You're not causing your body to adapt to the stress and stimulus of exercise which results in repair and growth.

Success Factor #2: Work Hard

If you want to change your body, you'll have to make an effort that takes you outside your comfort zone. You have to look forward to the workout being over. The intensity and the quality of the strain in your workout is what causes your brain to adapt and compensate for the physical stress that you're imposing upon your body.

It's not the specific exercises or different routines that get the results. It's working hard and consistently with simple, effective movements. I've seen countless men and women get very fit with extremely basic exercise routines. The key is that they pushed themselves.

Success Factor #3: Follow the Eating and Exercise Plan Correctly

How many times in your life have you performed poorly because you failed to follow the instructions correctly? It's like buying something that needs assembly. You put it together without reading the instructions and have unused parts left over. And then you wonder why it didn't work.

For you to be successful in your physical fitness endeavor, you're going to have to follow a plan that has proved itself again and again. Stay the course and don't deviate from one strategy to another if you want to get results. There are a lot of excellent philosophies in achieving physical fitness. If you don't like this one, choose another and stick with it.

Success Factor #4: Have Fun

Developing a physical fitness plan is not an exact science. There is room for a lot of artistic expression and personal style in how you exercise. There are many different ways to build a mousetrap. I like what King Solomon says in Ecclesiastes 11:9–10:

> Young man, it's wonderful to be young! Enjoy every minute of it. Do everything you want to do; take it all in. But remember that you must give an account to God for everything you do. So banish grief and pain.

Success Factor #5: Vary Your Workouts

The Lord created the human body to adapt to stresses that are imposed upon its systems. Once this adaptation takes place, these stresses become routine. Once your body adapts to your workouts, it stops progressing and begins to stagnate.

Even though it's important to be consistent with exercise, it's also important to change your workouts slightly every four to six weeks. This slight change is called variance. The idea is to keep your body in a constant state of progressive adaptation. You can vary your workouts by changing the order of your exercise. Or you can change the amount of weight you're lifting and the number of repetitions that you perform in each set of exercise.

"Keep stirring the pot, making your workouts fresh and interesting."

Variance can mean that you come up with new exercises to train certain areas of your body. The Lord created your body to have its own intelligence. It will tell you what it is craving in terms of movement and expression.

For aerobic exercise of your heart, lungs, and circulatory pathways, we use cross-training to overcome stale and routine exercise programs. Cross-training means changing your movement from, let's say, fitness walking to bicycling. Or it may mean adding in an occasional lap-swimming workout. Keep stirring the pot, making your workouts fresh and interesting. You never want to become bored with your workouts.

Success Factor #6: Listen to Your Body

Because your body has its own intelligence, not only will it tell you the type of exercise it wants; it will also tell you when you're doing too much. Muscle soreness and joint stiffness are to be expected when you first start exercising. In fact, advanced exercisers seek muscle soreness as a way of gauging the effectiveness of their training. However, there's a point where soreness can indicate you're doing too much in too short of a period of time. When this happens, the risk of injury increases. As a rule of thumb, if your body is tired, sore, and aches after your exercise but recovers by the time you're ready for your next workout, you're all right. But if you feel a focused, jabbing pain during a movement, this probably indicates you've injured that area to some extent.

This doesn't mean you should stop exercising. It means you should stop those movements that caused the jabbing pain until the pain goes away and the body adapts and heals. We call this *working out around* an injury. This is standard operating procedure for seasoned exercisers, but please do seek medical attention if you need it.

By the way, many orthopedic surgeons agree you should limit the duration of your workouts to one hour. Studies have shown that even moderate exercise can be overly traumatic if it lasts much more than sixty minutes. However, most exercise experts also agree that if you're not fatigued and ready for rest after an hour, you're probably not pushing yourself hard enough.

An hour of concentrated, methodical exercise is comparable to working eight hours of manual labor. After all, a manual laborer doesn't perform continuous sets and repetitions of a given movement. His work is performed on and off over the course of his workday.

Success Factor #7: Plan for the Long Haul

Remember, the Lord created your body to adapt to what you do over time. Do not look for instant results. Your primary motivation is for the long term: giving your body to God for his honor, glory, and purpose in your life. Matthew 6:33 says, "Seek first the kingdom of God and his righteousness, and all these things shall be added to you" (NKJV). Some of "these things" include the changes that happen to you physically, mentally, socially, and emotionally.

Look at your physical fitness as a journey, not a destination. I've been formally exercising for over fifty years now, and I still haven't arrived at the pinnacle of my physical fitness. The pinnacle would be to be without defect. You and I will never be without defect until we're with the Lord in our new bodies.

So, are you ready to get moving? Let's take a look at how to structure a day of physical fitness activity.

Your Timeline to Fitness

I get really excited when discussing the timeline for someone aspiring to a high degree of physical fitness because having a timeline gives people hope in a tangible way. It takes away the ambiguity when you see how long it takes to get physically fit and what the landmarks are along the way. What can you expect to change within your body over time, and in how much time?

I'll cut to the chase. My experience within this field says that, for the most part, you will be close to 95 percent as physically fit as you can ever become in one year. For most of you who are reading this book, time is going by pretty fast. One year is like tomorrow, isn't it? As I write this book, I'm in my mid-fifties. Yet I think of myself as a young man in my mid-twenties! It's so very strange to realize, especially when I see a reflection of myself, that I really am fifty-four. I thank God that I know I'm going to live forever, and that this body is only temporary. I am grateful for it, but I'm really looking forward to the new, improved model I'm going to receive.

Yet one year in the natural is still just one year. So, the idea that you can turn your body around and become revitalized in one year is a leap-for-joy realization. Take a look at figure 6.1.

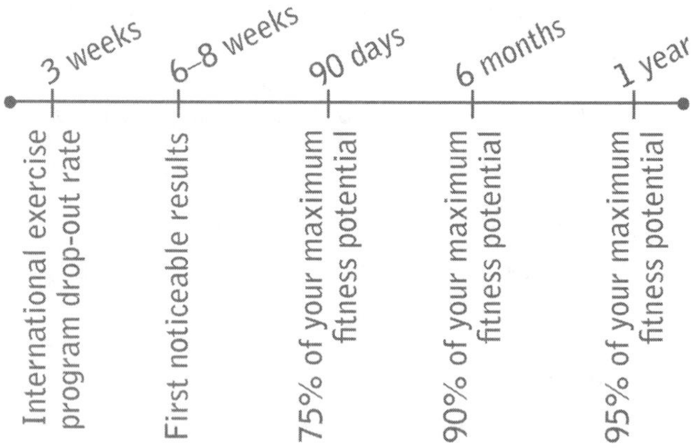

Figure 6.1 Timeline to physical fitness

I've taken great pleasure in designing and working with people in exercise programs since 1971. It didn't take me long to come to the realization that most people who begin a fitness program fail after only three weeks. I know that by now you've heard we live in a fast-food, fast-everything world. We want what we want right now! We're in such a hurry to get something or somewhere that, when we're stopped in traffic, we feel like driving up the muffler of the auto in front of us and down its radiator. The need for immediate gratification has become pandemic, especially in America.

Six to Eight Weeks

When I first start working with someone as a personal trainer, the first thing that I tell them is not to expect to lose any body mass for at least six to eight weeks. You can weigh yourself once a week on Friday morning, but that's it. If you lose some weight, great! But we're in this for the long haul, right? And our real motivation should be to honor God with our body, and not to be "buff with the stuff."

The reason that you will probably not lose any weight for six to eight weeks is that as you impose physical stress on your body, your remarkable brain immediately begins adapting to that stress. So as you condition your heart, lungs, and circulatory pathways, your blood and lymph fluid volumes *increase* as a result of the increased oxygen and nutrient demand. As you work to strengthen and tone the muscles, bones, and connective tissue, your body responds by *increasing* its durability and cross-sectional collagen thickness and content. The muscles of your body are 75 percent water. As you work your muscles on a consistent basis, they enlarge with *even more water* for improved function and muscle tone. Your joints act as sponges as you move your body in exercise. The joints increase in elasticity, suppleness, and mobility as they *increase* their fluid. I get so excited when I think of the marvel of how God created us. Right now, go to your Bible and read Psalm 139:13–18. We are wondrously made!

"Right now, go to your Bible and read Psalm 139:13-18. We are wondrously made!"

So the main reason you may not lose weight for a couple of months is, you're "building the house." Your body is under construction. It needs two-by-fours, nails, shingles, and glue, and it takes weight in the form of lean body mass to do this. In fact, I've had people who've actually gained weight. But I guarantee that your body fat percentage will have gone down substantially during this rebuilding process. I will also predict that your body will change in all the right places. Your clothes are going to fit looser and tighter in all the right places. Trust this process as your body transforms itself into what the Lord made it to be. Relax and be patient.

Ninety Days

This process of building lean body mass at the expense of your body fat will continue for six to twelve weeks. As you near the three-month mark, it will finally begin to normalize. You will have achieved approximately 75 percent of your genetic maximum in physical fitness. Think of it! In only ninety days, you're three quarters of the way there!

It's at this point where you will finally begin to lose unnecessary body mass. This body mass will remarkably be a combination of nonfunctional lean mass that you no longer need and the continual decrease in excess body fat percentage from throughout your body. Your muscles will increase in density and compactness as body fat is burned. Your stored fat on the outside layers of your skin will decrease and thin, showing an increase in your muscularity and definition. You'll start to see aspects of your body that you never knew you had, and because of this phenomenon, your motivation to press on will become even greater. If you've stuck it out for ninety days, you've got it!

Six Months

From ninety days to six months, your transformation and metamorphosis continues. However, the rate of perceived and actual change will slow down significantly. At six months, you'll be chiseled and svelte in your appearance. Your entire movement and countenance will be different. Friends and acquaintances that you haven't seen in a while will be shocked at the change in your appearance. They'll say, "You look great!" In six months, you're 90 percent of the way to being as physically fit as you'll ever be.

One Year

After six months of commitment to improving your physical fitness for the Lord's purpose in your life, it will now be part of who you are. Physical fitness will be an integrated part of your being. You will stay fit and eat right as a matter of course. This new you will be the standard operating procedure you live by. Healthy habits will have replaced destructive ones.

From six months to one year, you will settle into the business at hand, focusing your efforts on becoming what the Lord wants you to be and what he wants you to do—your mission. After one year of devotion to physical fitness, you will be 95 percent of what you will ever be. In some ways, you will be even fitter than you were when you were younger.

I can honestly say that at the age of fifty-four my fitness is greater than when I was in my prime at twenty-three. I weigh the same. But, if you saw a picture of me in a swimsuit now and compared it to a similar picture at age twenty-three, in many ways I look better. My body has continued to make improvements for thirty years. And the Lord isn't finished improving me. The most important time to get physically fit is as you get older. Of course, this goes for any and all learning and development.

Your New Physical Fitness Lifestyle

So, let's take a look at the plan for your new lifestyle. Here's what you'll want to strive for. Remember, talk with your doctor about beginning your new exercise program.

- Condition your heart, lungs, and circulatory pathways through aerobic exercise twenty to sixty minutes, five to six days per week.

- Condition your bones, joints, and muscles two to six days per week.
- Improve your body's flexibility and elasticity by conditioning five to six days per week.
- Reduce and maintain a lower body fat percentage 24/7 through consistent exercise and proper nutrition.
- Supply your body with the highest form of nutrients by choosing and ingesting whole, live, and raw foods when possible.
- Get at least seven to nine hours of sleep per night to maximize your recovery.
- Don't worry, be happy. Have joy, because this is what the Lord wants for your life as you serve him.

Okay, now we're ready to incorporate these components into the weekly model. First, take a look at figure 6.2.

Two-a-Days

This sounds like sports training practice from high school or college where you had to do the classic "two-a-days" to get ready for the season. Actually, I want you to have shorter but more frequent exercise workouts. As we'll discuss later, the key to increasing your metabolic rate is in *eating* and *moving* throughout your fifteen to seventeen hours of wakefulness.

You're probably wondering about the two aerobic workouts that I'm advocating on Tuesday, Thursday, and Saturday. *Aerobic* ("with oxygen") exercise is generally considered any low- to medium-intensity activity that you can sustain for a period of time. It forces your lungs to work, so it increases your cardiovascular endurance and also burns body fat. Examples would be walking, jogging, cycling, swimming. You should aim for twenty to sixty minutes of aerobic exercise five to six days per week. It is better to have two thirty-minute aerobic workouts at separate times during the day than to have one sixty-minute workout. The two shorter workouts will get your body systems ramped up each time, using an incredible amount of fuel, especially carbohydrates.

Day of the Week	Morning Workout	Afternoon Workout
Monday	Anaerobic	Aerobic
Tuesday	Aerobic	Aerobic
Wednesday	Anaerobic	Aerobic
Thursday	Aerobic	Aerobic
Friday	Anaerobic	Aerobic
Saturday	Aerobic	Aerobic
Sunday	The Lord's day is for fellowship, rest, and growth	

Figure 6.2 Weekly exercise schedule

Note: Depending on your church denomination, you may take Saturday as your Sabbath instead of Sunday. It makes no difference. Just adjust the model according to your needs.

Anaerobic Resistance Workouts

You'll see in the weekly model that a beginner performs resistance, or anaerobic, training workouts three days per week on an every-other-day basis. Resistance exercise is called *anaerobic,* meaning "without oxygen." It primarily burns sugar (carbohydrate) and uses all of the available oxygen in your nerves and muscles in that movement within sixty seconds. Anaerobic activity is performed at an intensity that cannot be sustained much longer than those sixty seconds. The benefits include increased muscle mass, strength, and speed, as well as fat-burning. Examples of anaerobic exercise would be sprints, jump rope, and weight-lifting.

Split Routines

I want you to graduate and ease into your workouts. Of course, I believe that a four-day-split routine of resistance conditioning is better than a three day schedule. By adding a fourth day, you'll increase your strength and muscle toning by an additional 25 percent. You need the fourth day to do a comprehensive job in your bone, joint, and muscle conditioning. Three days is good, but four days is better. The four-day-split routine resistance workout looks like this: You work your upper body on Monday and Thursday, and your lower body on Tuesday and Friday. Or, you could start Mondays with your lower body. It really doesn't matter that much. Then, Wednesday and Saturday could be aerobic only.

You might be wondering if five or six days of anaerobic resistance conditioning would be better than the four-day-split routine. Not really. In fact, unless you're an advanced exerciser who wants to do bodybuilding, the additional strength workouts will actually take away from your fitness development. I'd rather have to do a couple of anaerobic sprint workouts, whether running, swimming, or bicycling, than lift weights for a fifth or sixth day in my week. We'll discuss sprints in an upcoming chapter. But I will say again that, to me, sprints are church!

tip: Eat and Move

When is the last time you had a stalk of celery with some old fashioned peanut butter on it? Have one now! I love the snap and crunch of eating this fun, delicious, and nutritious snack.

EAT AND MOVE:

KICK START YOUR METABOLISM

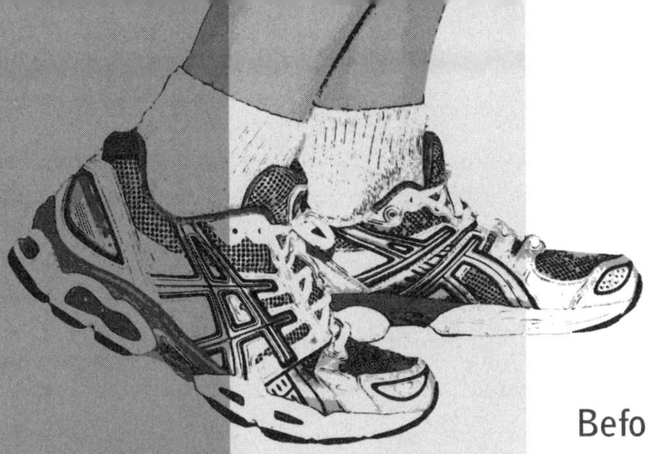

7

Before we look further into physical fitness, I need to explain that we want to maximize your genetic potential. This concept is called *thermogenesis,* which is the body's production of heat and energy. The two ways we produce energy are by eating and moving. If you increase the frequency of eating and moving throughout your day, you will increase the rate at which this heat and energy is utilized.

The rate at which you use your energy is called *metabolism.* Metabolism is highly genetically determined and also affected by your gender, size, age, and activity level. Some people have a very high metabolism that allows them to eat a large quantity of food per day yet stay slim and trim. Some people have a very low metabolism; if they eat a moderate amount, they become overweight. Most of us fall somewhere in the middle of these two extremes.

No matter what your genetic metabolic rate is, it can be increased to utilize and burn more of the calories you ingest at a higher rate. The strategy is a combination of meal and exercise frequency. In figure 7.1 I've provided you with a thermogenic day-at-a-glance so that you can see how this concept plays out in your waking hours in a 24-hour day. I'm going to talk you through this now.

Pre-morning Exercise Preparation

First you wake up, hopefully after seven to nine hours of quality sleep. Eat a light or mini breakfast before doing a resistance (or weight training) workout. You'll need to get your blood sugar level up before you exercise intensely. Otherwise, shortly into your workout you'll feel weak and possibly sick to your stomach. When you exercise to the point that you have to stop and rest, it means your nerves and muscles have run out of oxygen. This oxygen debt can result in the increase of lactic acid, producing nausea. A light breakfast could be a slice of whole grain toast with some nut butter on it, or it could be a small bowl of cereal and milk, or maybe a fruit smoothie.

Morning	1. Wake up after 7–9 hours of quality sleep. 2. Pre-morning exercise preparation. 3. Do your morning workout. 4. Eat breakfast like a king. 5. Perform your morning activities. 6. Optional pre-lunch aerobic workout. 7. Eat a queen-sized lunch. One o'clock rule—No starch! 70% of daily calories are consumed.
Afternoon	8. Perform your afternoon activities. 9. Do your pre-dinner primary aerobic workout. 10. Eat dinner like a pauper.
Evening	11. Digest, relax, and enjoy relationships. 12. If hungry, have an evening snack. 13. Prepare for a great night's sleep.

Figure 7.1 The thermogenic training concept

Don't eat anything before doing an aerobic workout in the morning. Your aerobic workout conditions your heart, lungs, and circulatory pathways. You should do it at an intensity that allows you to continue moving for an extended period of time without having to rest and recover. Aerobic exercise burns body fat. By not eating before this type of workout, you force your body to go into fat-burning mode sooner. In any type of exercise, the first twelve to fifteen minutes of movement primarily is burning sugar from your body, even if the intensity is low.

Do Your Morning Workout

As mentioned in the previous chapter, resistance exercise is called *anaerobic,* meaning "without oxygen." Anaerobic workouts, such as weight training or running sprints, should have a maximum duration of forty-five to sixty seconds per repetition.

On the other hand, if you're doing a morning aerobic training, go from twenty to sixty minutes, as explained earlier.

Eat Breakfast like a King

Your metabolic rate is highest in the morning. And when you exercise in the morning, it increases your natural metabolic rate. So the largest meal of your day should be breakfast, especially after morning exercise. Whether you've performed an aerobic or anaerobic workout, your body is screaming for fuel and nutrients, the building blocks to repair your body from the stress it has just endured.

"A light breakfast could be a slice of whole grain toast with some nut butter on it, or it could be a small bowl of cereal and milk, or maybe a fruit smoothie."

Now is the time to enjoy higher calorie and higher fat foods, when your body's rate of burning calories is at its highest. If you're going to eat foods like pancakes or pie or cake, breakfast is the time to do it. Breakfast can include breads; eggs; lean protein sources such as red meat, fish, and poultry; dairy products such as milk and yogurt; and fibrous fruits such as berries and bananas.

In Ecclesiastes 9:7, King Solomon says, "So go ahead. Eat your food and drink…with a happy heart, for God approves of this."

By the way, if you have to get to work before you can eat this king-sized meal, you may have to brown-bag it. You may have to eat on the way to work, or right after you safely arrive. But please be careful if you're driving an automobile!

Perform Your Morning Activities

Once your body's metabolic rate has been ramped up from bouts of eating and exercise, you're ready to tackle your morning work with terrific vitality. Talk about productivity—wow!

If you get hungry before lunch, be sure to have nutritious snacks such as fresh fruit, nuts, or seeds with you at all times. You don't want to get caught with no food available when you're hungry. If you're hungry for too long a period of time, your body will start to ingest its own lean body mass of organ, muscle, and bone tissue. You should be eating every two to three hours. This is the concept of meal frequency. A small meal is one hundred to four hundred calories. Eating an apple, for example, would be considered a small meal.

Optional Pre-lunch Aerobic Workout

Most of the research on the body's daily circadian rhythms suggests that our highest energy level for the day is around eleven in the morning. So, if you have the time, you may want to get another thermogenic exercise in before you eat lunch. Ideally, you could go for a twenty- to thirty-minute power walk. But even a few minutes of some form of exercise would elevate your rate of burning calories.

One of the most important keys to improving your physical fitness is taking advantage of exercise opportunities whenever possible. Decide to develop a physical fitness attitude, eating and exercising in small increments throughout your day. If you do this, you'll become incredibly fit in a relatively short period of time.

Eat a Queen-sized Lunch

Lunch time is generally between eleven and one anywhere in the world. Sadly, for a majority of people, this is their first meal of the day. The tragedy is that they have not supplied their body with the fuel and nutrients it needs when it needs them the most. Their bodies probably ingested significant amounts of their lean body mass to supply their body's energy needs.

However, for the person who has adopted a healthy thermogenic routine, lunch is still a fairly large meal. Depending on how high you increased your metabolic rate through your morning exercise workout and your morning work activities, you may be really hungry for lunch.

So go ahead and enjoy a substantial meal. However, because your body's energy needs have been largely supplied in the morning, I recommend that you become aware of the amount of starchy carbohydrates you consume in your day, starting with lunch. Starch is considered a super sugar. It's found in grains, cereals, flour, rice, pasta, noodles, potatoes, and chips. If you're trying to lose weight, start minimizing the amount of starch you eat at lunch. You might decide to have only one slice of bread in a sandwich, for example. Instead of a bag of chips, have a bowl of soup, a salad, or a piece of fruit. Remember, whatever calories your body cannot utilize metabolically at that moment will be stored as fat.

One of the strategies I have used successfully with my clients is what I call the One O'clock Rule: they cannot eat any starch after 1:00 PM. This is actually very forgiving because they can eat as much starchy food as they want before that time. So, if you're hungry for spaghetti, have it by lunch.

The Russians have performed more research on exercise and human performance than anyone else in history. They say 70 percent of our daily calories should be consumed by lunch.

Afternoon Activities

If you've ever had to speak before a group of people after lunch, you know how difficult it is for both yourself and the people who are trying to listen to you. The Lord has created within the human body a secondary drop in body temperature and energy that occurs between one and four in the afternoon. Many cultures have embraced this reality by taking a siesta during this time of day, then working into the evening. North American culture attempts to fight our biology and maintain a work schedule. But a well-placed nap of twenty to sixty minutes can do wonders to restore our energy and vitality for the rest of our activities.

The Pre-dinner Primary Aerobic Workout

By four in the afternoon, the human body cycles back to a higher thermal temperature and potential energy output. So the best time to do your primary aerobic workout, which cleans out the gunk from your arteries and other blood vessels, is at the end of your stress-packed day but before your dinner. Of course, the best time for you to do any type of exercise is when you can. Everyone's life is so unique that *when* you can exercise supersedes "the best time to exercise" philosophy.

If you can aerobically exercise forty to (at most) sixty minutes before your last major meal, it increases your body's ability to digest dinner, and even helps prepare you to emotionally and mentally relax for your evening with friends and family. Also, at this time of day, any form of exercise will suppress your appetite, making you less likely to overeat.

Eat Dinner like a Pauper

Most people agree that dinner is the most important meal to share with others. There are those people who still consider "breaking bread" with someone as establishing a covenant of sorts. In any case, you'll probably often eat dinner with family and friends. However, dinner should be considered the smallest of your major meals. It is still important, though, that you eat enough food so that you're no longer hungry. Dinner should include a lean complete protein source such as fish, poultry, or red meat, with fibrous vegetables such as mixed greens, peas, broccoli, cauliflower, or carrots. By this time of the day it's prudent to keep starches such as bread, pasta, and chips to a minimum.

The Evening Snack

Please don't go to bed hungry. Not only will your sleep suffer, but you will also deprive your body of the nutrients it needs for processes it performs while you are sleeping.

Remember, if you're hungry a couple of hours before bedtime, your body is demanding food. Go ahead and eat something, but be careful not to eat past your hunger level. An evening snack could be a cup of yogurt, a glass of low-fat milk, a small fruit smoothie, organic ice cream, or an easy-to-digest piece of fruit, such as a banana or strawberries. You should be aware of what causes you indigestion by this point in your life. You will sleep poorly if you have indigestion, so use common sense and avoid those foods before going to bed.

Before I close this chapter, I want you to look at an illustration that will give you a better idea of what the thermogenic events of eating and moving should look like throughout your day.

You can see from figure 7.2 that every time you eat or exercise, your metabolic rate ramps back up. If you increase these thermogenic events throughout your waking hours, you will use significantly more energy. This is how to improve the function of every system in your body, increase lean body mass, and decrease body fat.

tip: Eat and Move

How about a set of pushups? Start on the ground or place your hands shoulder-width apart on a bench or wall. With your midsection and back straight like a plank, lower your body to the ground or surface. Keep your head and neck in line with your spine as you perform as many quality pushups as you can. You'll feel great afterward!

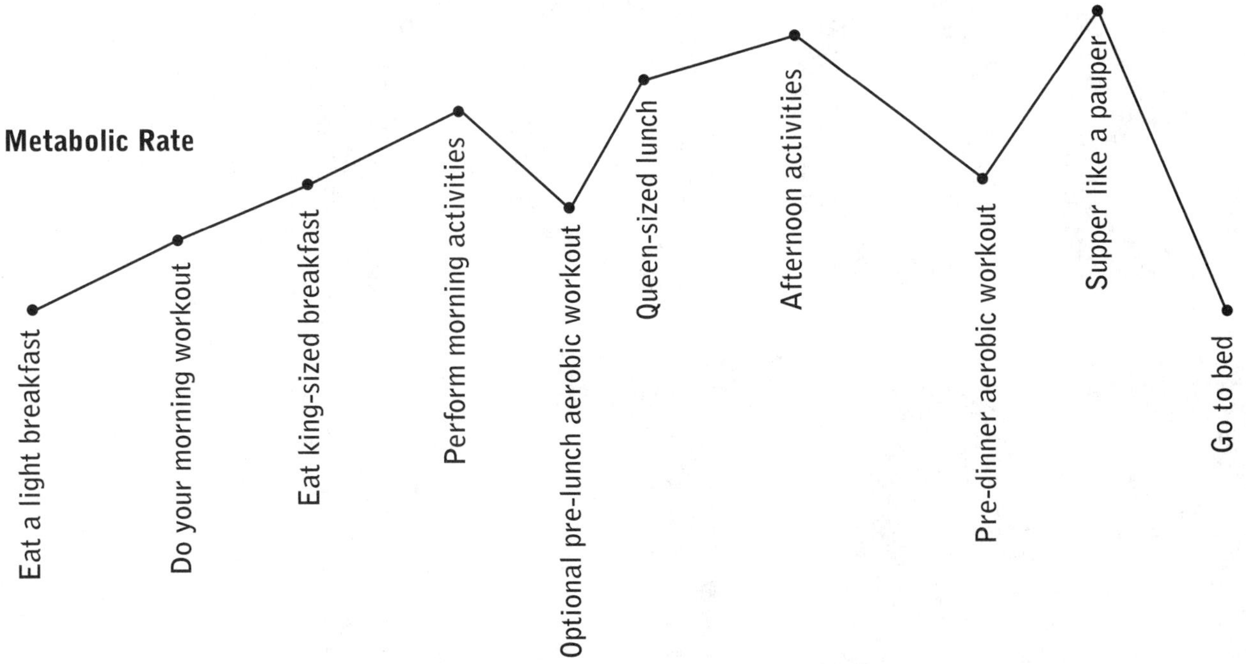

FIGURE 7.2 THERMOGENESIS: CREATION OF HEAT AND ENERGY

GET BALANCED: REDUCE YOUR BODY FAT

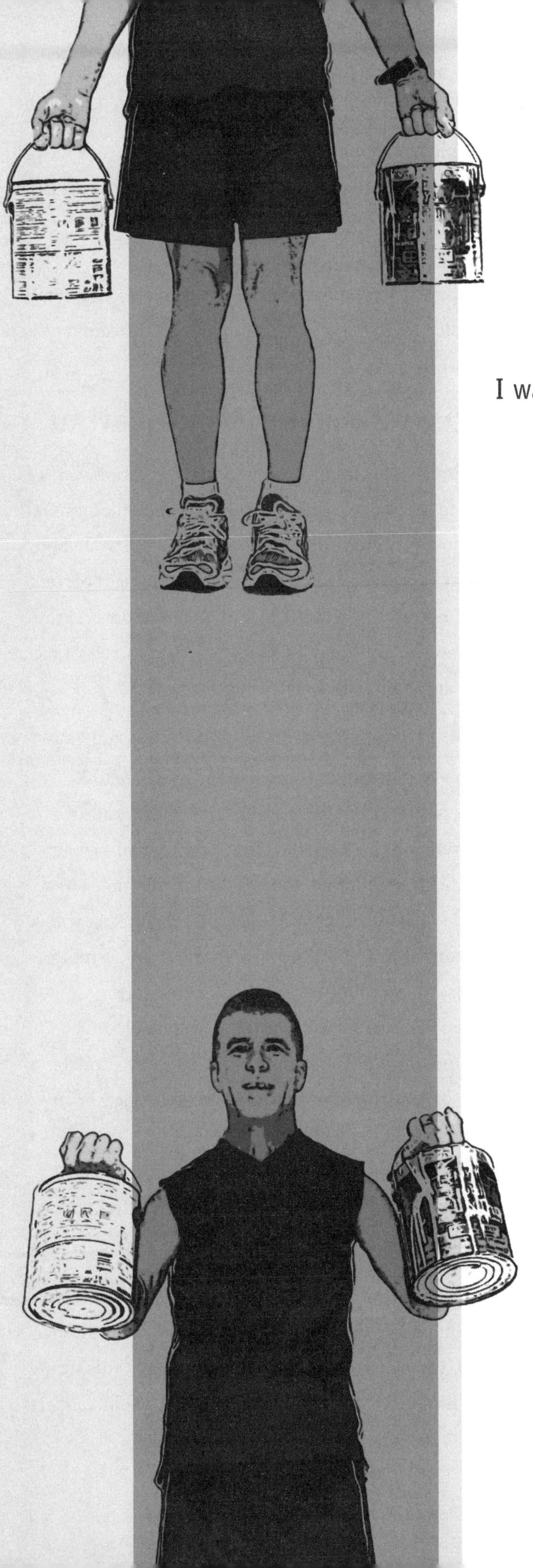

8

I was a fat kid growing up. People who know me are shocked to hear me share that part of my past. I was also very fit in terms of my muscular-skeletal strength and joint flexibility. But I didn't invest enough time in aerobic conditioning as I should have. My eating habits were completely unrestrained. I had no concept of what overeating meant. I loved desserts. I could easily eat dessert first and then the rest of my meal. My favorites included banana cream pie, peanut butter and chocolate rice-crispy bars, and my mother's famous fudge brownies. I did eat the good stuff, too. I ate everything—too much of everything.

My high exercise output kept me from becoming medically obese, but I was chubby. The "fat" comments from my peers hurt my feelings, but obviously not enough to motivate me. By the time I got to college, I had had enough. I knew what to do, and I did it. I never believed in diets, even though my mother went on almost every one imaginable. Don't get me wrong. My mother was an attractive woman, but she battled excess body fat as well.

Other than right after the time of my running injury (discussed in the epilogue), I've never again been overweight since I was twenty years old. I feel my best and the closest to the Lord when I'm at my leanest. I really love that tight, empty feeling within my body. An orthopedic surgeon friend described me as looking "close to the bone." To me, it was a great compliment. Even though I wasn't a Christian during my fat years, I didn't eat from emotion or distress. I just loved food! It hadn't become an idol to me; it was just out of balance with the other components in my life.

I think Jesus must have enjoyed eating good food. After all, he made the ingredients for all of it. The four Gospels illustrate events where Jesus was eating with or feeding others. It's interesting that when Jesus was tempted by Satan in the wilderness, food was the first thing Satan threw at him. And, of course, we see the Lord's reply in Matthew 4:4, where Jesus says, "People need more than bread for their life; they must feed on every word of God." Most people know that gluttony is immoral and goes directly against the laws of nature. We are at a historic point here in America where two-thirds of our citizens are considered overweight. Two-thirds! However, it's not entirely their fault. Who are the real culprits? I don't know, but the food industry does not always act in the best interests of the consumer. The food industry in the United States cares about making food taste the best it can at the lowest possible cost. Are they intentionally genetically altering soybeans, corn, and wheat to hurt us? I really don't think so. Are they loading foods, vitamins, and supplements with preservatives, additives, and colored dyes to cause us disease? I don't know. All I know is, this is what they are doing. As Christians, we have much more important things to focus on than what the world is doing in this area. We do, however, have to be aware of what is really happening and take personal responsibility for our health through proper exercise and nutrition. By the way, daily exercise is the best way to buy yourself some time while you're figuring out how to reduce your body fat and detoxify yourself.

One of the laws of nature the Lord created was for body fat to encapsulate any poison or toxin in the body. Because we're consuming more poison than ever before, the body fat levels of our people are continuing to rise unchecked. The problem is, people don't know what's in the food they're eating. You can't keep eating genetically altered and hormone-infused food without bad things beginning to happen to you. Excess body fat is now recognized as a primary risk factor for coronary heart disease, cancer, diabetes, and joint injuries. After all, the leanest animals live the longest. We need to wake up!

Okay, I'll stop preaching. The rest of this chapter is dedicated to giving you an action plan to get lean.

Eating-Behavior Modification

The Lord created hunger pangs for us to become aware of when to eat and when to stop eating. This is the simplest but most profound strategy to help you get your body back to its ideal balance. This balance is the right percentage of body fat in relation to your lean body mass. Your body needs fat to function at its best. As a matter of fact, body fat provides four major benefits:

- It is the transportation system for important hormone regulators and the vitamins A, E, D, and K.
- The skin layer of fat protects your body from the extremes of heat and cold. You'll notice that as your body fat level drops, you will be much more sensitive to cold weather and water temperature. As you become leaner, your body will also become more efficient at cooling itself in hot temperatures.
- Deep internal fat protects your vulnerable organs from injury if you are involved in some kind of fall or experience impact to your body, such as an automobile accident.
- Body fat acts as fuel for your body's energy needs during low to moderate movement intensities, such as in aerobic fitness walking.

So, what is the ideal percentage of body fat to be physically fit? I can give you the percentages, but, unfortunately, the means of accurately and reliably measuring body fat percentage is not available. Skin-fold calipers and electrical impedance devices are not dependable. The only definitive test is called a DEXA scan (double x-ray). This is a $75,000 machine, and only a few organizations even have them.

In all of my thirty-eight years of experience in the physical fitness field, I've come to believe that the best indicator of body fat/lean body mass balance is the Body Mass Index. Check online for a free, easy way to calculate yours. For example, I'm five foot seven (sixty-seven inches) and weigh 137 pounds. According to the Body Mass Index I'm right in the middle of my acceptable body weight. I have a small to medium bone frame, so I could be a few pounds lighter and still have a lean but physically fit body fat percentage. The good news is, as long as you're within your parameter, that's close enough. Look at what it says in Deuteronomy 32:15:

> But Israel soon became fat and unruly; the people grew heavy, plump, and stuffed! Then they abandoned the God who had made them; they made light of the Rock of their salvation.

I encourage you to get your body fat and body mass in balance for the Lord. If you do, he will bless you for your diligence.

Anyway, let's get back to hunger pangs. The feeling of hunger is your body's way of telling you it needs fuel. You have about a thirty- to sixty-minute window of time to satisfy this need before your brain starts breaking down your own lean body mass to supply the necessary energy. You need to plan ahead and have an assortment of healthy food with you at all times, preferably in an airtight cooler.

"We have to take take personal responsibility for our health through proper exercise and nutrition."

Before I give these seven eating guidelines, remember: they are *guidelines*, not laws. If you become legalistic about these, you will lose friends. You might even fail to go wherever the Lord is calling you, because you might have to eat food that isn't on our list. My attitude is do the best you can whenever you can.

Hunger Guidelines

1. With the exception of breakfast, only eat when you feel hungry, not according to the time of day. I know that you've heard about the importance of eating a healthy breakfast. Your metabolic rate and your need for fuel are at their highest in the morning. For many people, however, they don't feel hungry in the morning and don't eat anything until lunch. I want you to trust that if you make a point of eating breakfast, you will become hungry as you begin to eat. When you get into the positive habit of eating in the morning, your body will learn to be hungry at waking.

   Lunch and dinner are different, though. If it's lunchtime or dinnertime and you're not hungry, don't eat—even if everyone else is. This may seem socially uncomfortable at first, but people will come to understand and respect your motives. Of course, eating a meal with someone is for relationships, so sit down and be with them, even if you're not eating. Learn to eat only when you're hungry.
2. As you begin to eat because you're hungry, become aware of the moment you're no longer hungry. At

that point, you must stop eating, no matter how much food is still on your plate. Perform one of the toughest exercises of all—"pushaways."

The Lord made food taste so good that sometimes it's easy to keep eating out of appetite rather than real hunger. The danger of eating out of appetite or from emotional needs is that the fuel you've taken in is not needed and will be stored as excess body fat. So the seesaw of gaining and losing weight begins. Gaining and losing weight is very stressful on the systems of your body. Get rid of the unnecessary body fat and keep it off.

If you adapt this simple hunger-pang principle, you will become hungry every two to three hours. This creates the meal frequency concept that we referred to earlier. You will automatically begin eating five to six small- to moderate-volume meals every day, and as you read earlier, meal frequency is half of the thermogenic process—eat and move.

3. Most authorities recommend you drink at least eight, eight-ounce glasses of pure, filtered water every day—not to fill you up and suppress hunger, but to hydrate your body and provide the medium for proper digestion.
4. Consume 20 to 30 percent of your daily calories from fat. Most Western cultures consume over 40 percent of their calories from fat, primarily animal or saturated fat. Saturated or hydrogenated fat is solid at room temperature. This solid fat plugs up everything inside your body, most critically your blood passages, so here are a few things to remember.

   Only eat animal-source protein and fat according to your energy needs. I'll be discussing this in depth in the next chapter. Consume no more than four to seven ounces of red meat, fish, or poultry at a sitting. This is an amount that could fit in the palm of your hand. Bake, broil, or boil the meat that you cook. Stay away from deep frying in vegetable fat because vegetable oils are unstable at high temperatures, resulting in the creation of trans fats or unhealthy compounds like acrylamides. Microwaving your food has now become suspect, so limit it as a primary cooking alternative.
5. Stop eating genetically modified grains such as wheat, corn, and soybeans as much as possible. Also avoid growth-hormone-injected animal products. As mentioned earlier, your body will store fat in order to encapsulate these unnatural toxins.
6. Consistently do the daily and weekly exercise programs. This will keep your body revved up and your metabolism high.
7. Don't lose more than one to two pounds a week. If you lose more than two pounds in a week, most of your weight loss will be lean body mass, not body fat.

   I know that you or someone you know believes that they've lost multiple pounds in a single day. This type of weight loss is water weight, not body fat. To lose even one pound requires a deficit of 3,500 calories. This is a significant amount of calories to consume or burn off in a 24-hour period and, for most people, is highly unlikely, no matter what they're doing.

The principles I've shared in this chapter will not only reduce your excess body fat. These same strategies will also help you bring down your blood pressure and cholesterol levels. They may also help you lower the dosage of your medications or stop needing them altogether.

As we close this chapter, remember: You will succeed if you commit for the long haul in your physical fitness development. Do it for the Lord, to obey and honor him, not to seek quick fixes. Your excess body fat and body weight will normalize over time. Remember the timeline we're working on. The Lord will bless you for your perseverance and determination.

tip: Eat and Move

Act like a rabbit and enjoy some organic baby carrots. Eat about five to seven of these vitamin A and beta-carotene-loaded powerhouses.

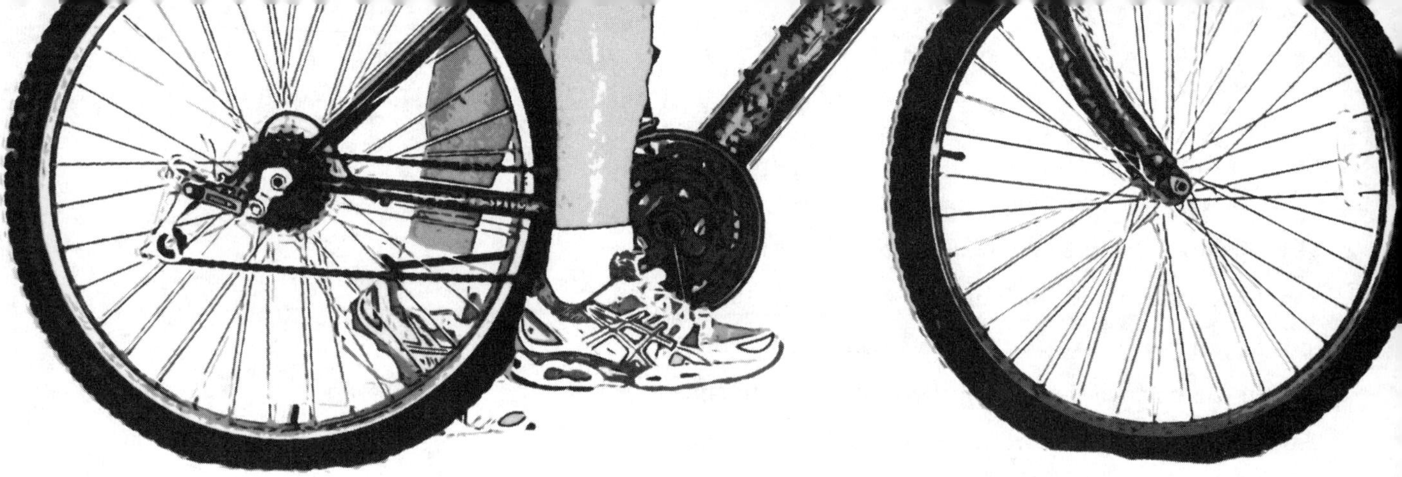

GET HEALTHY:
REALISTIC NUTRITION

9

My wife Rebecca and I often say that "a person's unique perception is his reality." Nowhere is this more applicable than in the very controversial area of nutrition. What people consider nutritious food is relative. One person's moderation is another person's extreme.

Back in the early 1980s, I was training a 185-pound state wrestling champion from Wisconsin. One day I happened to see him at the local grocery store having lunch. His lunch was chocolate éclair pastries and a quart of chocolate milk. Yet this eighteen-year-old young man was lean, muscular, and had the body of a mythical Greek god! How can that be? The answer lies in the physical nature of youth. The human male does not stop developing to his full potential until around the age of twenty-five. Females reach their full potential a few years earlier. The Lord created the human body so that, as long as there is a growth demand on its systems, it can make the most of whatever quality of nutrients it's receiving. This is the same concept as to why morning is the best time to eat your goodies—the less nutritious foods. Your metabolic rate is at its highest in the morning, but it will gradually slow down right up to the time you are ready to sleep for the night.

This is similar to the way your metabolic rate operates over the course of your life. As the years go by, your metabolic rate gradually decreases, no matter what your genetics are. I'm sure that my young wrestler, who is now in his early forties, is either extremely overweight or has adjusted his eating habits. So, as the human body ages, consistent, quality exercise and eating the most nutritious foods become more and more important. By the way, this principle is valid for mental exercise as well. The older we get, the more we should be committed to learning new things, to keep mentally fit.

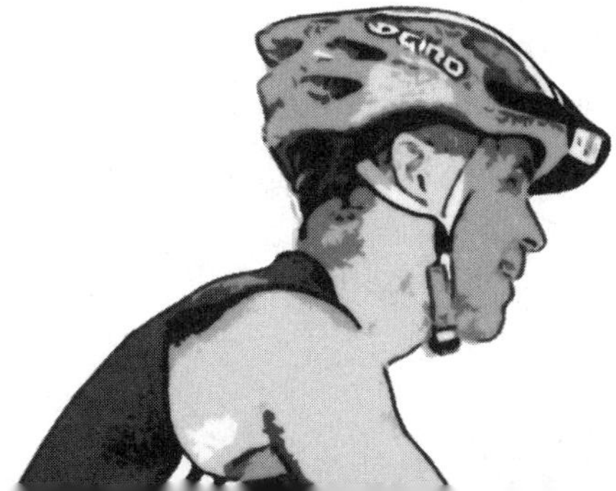

I called this chapter "realistic nutrition" because, for most people, our habits have to be close enough to the ideal to be effective but also practical. Obsessive people say, "I don't eat that" or "I can't have that." These folks are difficult to be around and are definitely no fun. A proper nutritional lifestyle has to be forgiving to be attainable. Realistic also means that it has to be affordable and available, no matter where you are in the world.

Proper Nutrition Defined

So, here's my definition of proper nutrition. Proper nutrition is choosing food to eat that is as high in energy value, minerals, vitamins, and fiber as possible. Food should be nutritionally dense, that is, have a high ratio of nutrients per calorie. With that in mind, what choice is more nutritious: a cream-filled, white-flour, white-sugar cake, or an organic apple? You get the point. Of course, depending on the circumstances, pickings might be slim. You have to make the most of what you have available.

My goal is to educate you so that you will be empowered to make the right eating choices. Let's start with some easy-to-understand guidelines listed in Figure 9.1.

This list of guidelines we've just seen is not exhaustive. But it will give you a great start. Now, let's take a deeper look at the primary food fuels.

Carbohydrates

Carbohydrates are various types of sugar molecules that the body breaks down into glucose, which is the primary fuel on which your body runs. Carbohydrates appear as sugars, fibers, and starches. Your body will even break down protein and fat into sugar, if necessary. Fruits, vegetables, grains, and beans give you your carbohydrates. How quickly the body converts any carbohydrate into glucose (a process which affects blood sugar levels) is measured as the food's glycemic index. Complex carbohydrates, or those with a lower glycemic load, are generally broken down more steadily and evenly into the body's glucose fuel. This means energy supplied over a longer period, lower spike in blood sugar levels, and less likelihood of the body storing it as fat. Minimally processed, whole grains and beans and whole, raw, and unprocessed fruits and vegetables are your best choices. Try to avoid refined carbohydrates—those that are refined, bleached, and processed. They include white sugar, white flour, most fruit juices, candy bars, and most canned foods.

Depending on your energy needs, which are determined by your basal metabolic rate—that is, the minimum needed to regulate body temperature and perform basic body functions like breathing and circulation—(a rate affected by size, age, gender, and genetics) plus your activity level. Just remember to make sure that they're as whole, raw, and unprocessed as possible.

Proteins

Proteins are responsible for the repair and growth of your lean body mass. Your skin, muscles, organs, bones, hair, and nails are made of proteins synthesized from the amino acids in the protein you ingest.

Protein comes from two primary sources: animals and plants. Animal sources include red meat, such as beef, lamb, and venison. They also include seafood, such as freshwater and saltwater fish. Poultry such as chicken, turkey, duck, and pheasant are also animal sources of protein, as are eggs and dairy products. Plant proteins come from vegetables, seeds, nuts, and legumes. Plant proteins are incomplete proteins, meaning that they don't contain all the essential amino-acid building blocks in one complete package like animal proteins do. This is why vegetarians need to make sure that they balance their food choices to ensure that they end up with a protein combination that

1. Choose food that has the highest value in energy, vitamins, minerals, and fiber.
2. Choose raw, whole foods as often as possible (seeds, nuts, fruit, vegetables, grains).
3. Eat as much organically grown food as possible.
4. Limit or don't eat food that is genetically modified or injected with growth hormones.
5. Limit or don't eat food that has been sprayed with pesticides or enhanced with food additives, preservatives, or color dyes.
6. Limit or don't eat food high in saturated fat, white sugar, corn syrup, maltodextrin, refined flours, and food starches.
7. Limit or don't eat food that has been deep-fried in any kind of oil.
8. Limit or avoid altogether carbonated drinks. They're high in acid and will weaken your bones.
9. Eat whole-grain oats, rice, rye, and millet. Limit whole-grain wheat, corn, and soybeans.
10. Choose lean, complete protein sources: red meat, fish, poultry, and dairy (try to get free-range and grass-fed).
11. Eat cruciferous vegetables, such as brussels sprouts, cabbage, broccoli, and cauliflower.
12. Eat yellow and orange foods, such as squash, sweet potatoes, pumpkin, carrots, and apricots.
13. Eat green leafy vegetables, such as spinach, kale, romaine lettuce, mustard greens, turnip greens, and beet greens.
14. Consume small amounts of butter, and avoid margarine, even the supposedly healthy safflower and sunflower oil varieties.
15. Choose low-fat, organic dairy products. Be careful with raw milk until your body gets used to it.
16. For cooking, bake, broil, or boil your food. Go easy on microwaving and charbroiling.

Figure 9.1 Nutrition guidelines

will cover the bases of all nine essential amino acids. Eating a wide a variety of fruits, vegetables, seeds, and nuts is the key. A grain like rice plus a legume like black beans, for instance, makes a complete protein.

Like carbohydrates, your protein needs for lean body mass repair and growth will vary. If you're performing daily anaerobic resistance training, you will need more protein than someone who is not exercising, or someone who is only doing aerobics. Here's a good rule of thumb:

- Eat 20 to 30 percent of your daily calories from animal and plant protein sources.
- Eat 0.6 grams of protein per pound of body weight if you're not currently exercising.
- Eat 0.8 grams of protein per pound of body weight if you're doing resistance strength training two to three days per week.
- Eat one gram of protein per pound if you're resistance training four to six days per week.

This will seem like a lot of protein to ingest, and it will take some focused effort to accomplish. Remember to choose low-fat, organic sources of protein that are minimally processed and, if plant-based, uncooked if possible. Animal sources of protein have to be cooked to kill harmful bacteria. But don't burn the meat. Boiling, steaming, and stewing are the best ways to keep the nutrients within the food.

Fats

Fat is what gives food flavor. This is why people enjoy high-fat foods so much. Fat is the primary fuel source for extended low- to moderate-intensity energy needs. Like protein, fat is derived from animal and plant sources. All fats are some combination of saturated, monounsaturated, and polyunsaturated molecules. Animal fat is primarily a saturated fat. Because it is solid, we have to be careful how much we consume on a daily and weekly basis. Most experts agree that even heavy exercisers shouldn't consume more than five to seven meals a week from animal protein/fat sources. Most plant oils are polyunsaturated and/or monounsaturated. Polyunsaturated fat comes mainly from vegetables (like corn, soy, and safflower) and is largely liquid at room temperature. We should limit even polyunsaturated fat. Monounsaturated fat is a liquid fat that actually thins the blood and frees it of obstructions. Organic peanut butter, avocados, almonds, walnuts, macadamia nuts, and ripe olives are excellent sources of monounsaturated fat. Cooking with cold-pressed, extra virgin olive oil is a great way to prepare food. It makes food taste delicious and is healthy for you. My wife, Rebecca, even uses it every day as a skin lotion.

Again, like carbohydrates and proteins, your total fat intake will vary according to your body's energy needs. Consume 20 to 30 percent of your total daily calories from fat. The higher your energy needs, the higher your fat intake.

What and When to Eat

You may already know your body well enough to know when to eat the healthy foods that you enjoy. Let's discuss the *what* and *when* of eating.

Breakfast

Breakfast seems to be the best time to have your breads, cereals, and starchy carbohydrates, like potatoes. Breakfast is also the best time for you to have eggs and low-fat dairy products (that are raw and unpasteurized, if available). The reason for raw dairy is, the high heat in pasteurizing destroys significant amounts of amino acids, enzymes, and vitamins in the food. You will have to adapt to raw dairy products carefully and over time. Breakfast is also a natural time of the day to have fruit, such as cantaloupe, bananas, berries, and citrus. You may eat some meat at breakfast, such as turkey sausage or lean ground beef. If possible, try to secure organic, free-range, and grass-fed protein whenever possible. This should be your biggest meal of the day, so enjoy!

Lunch

For most people I know, lunch has become a time of eating on the fly—taking maybe fifteen minutes. I know a lot of people who eat lunch while they're driving or while they just keep on working. But I believe the Lord wants us to take pause, relax a bit, and regenerate at the middle of our day. You need to invest some time for lunch. This investment of time will pay you back in terms of renewed energy and mental focus for the rest of your day.

For Rebecca and me, lunch has now become our time to eat fibrous fruits, such as apples, pears, nectarines, plums, peaches, and bananas. We also enjoy pumpkin seeds, sunflower seeds, and raw almonds. Lunch used to be a time when we ate salads, soups, and whole-grain sandwiches with uncured, organic deli meats. But it seems that, for us, it takes a lot of time to properly digest this kind of food in the middle of the day. Develop a lunch plan that works best for your unique physiology, and that you can look forward to. Remember, this should be your "queen-sized" meal.

Dinner

The evening meal is where most people sit down, relax, and have time with their family and friends. This is also the meal that most people take time to think out and prepare. Preparation doesn't have to mean complexity, though. It does mean ensuring quality: nutritious, delicious food that is easy to digest and sets you up for a good night's sleep. Dinner is the time to have four to seven ounces of animal-source proteins (unless you're a vegetarian) and fibrous vegetables such as mixed greens, pea pods, broccoli, carrots, and cauliflower. Sometimes Rebecca will stir-fry these veggies all together with poultry or ground beef. Other times we just have a mixed salad with some cold-water fish such as tuna on some rice cakes.

Dinner should be your "pauper-sized" meal. It should also be a low-starch meal, because at this time of day your metabolic rate is getting really low and you can't justify the calories. If you're craving starch, prepare a small quantity of brown or wild rice, or have some corn on the cob. Sometimes Rebecca and I have some salsa with organic, blue corn chips. Dinner is the time to pay careful attention to when you feel full. Do not eat past your hunger.

Evening Snack

If you're following the thermogenic daily system I've described, you may be hungry a couple of hours before you go to bed. Don't go to bed hungry or you won't sleep well.

The evening snack should be a very small quantity of food that balances out protein, carbohydrates, and fats. If you have too much protein, it will keep you up. If you have too many carbs, your body will store them as fat. But then again, your body will also turn a predominantly protein food into fat if you have more than you can use. Whatever you have, consume just enough to take the edge off your hunger. Eat a couple of pieces, or a couple spoonfuls, or maybe a small handful of something. Here are a few ideas that we use with success:

- Have two pieces of organic dark chocolate that has at least 70 percent cacao content. It's delicious, has significant protein, and is high in antioxidants.
- Have a small glass of organic, low-fat milk, even chocolate. It's a perfect balance of protein, carbohydrate, and fat.
- Have a small yogurt fruit smoothie. This is a great snack because it also satisfies your sweet tooth.
- A small bowl of organic popcorn that is popped with an expeller-pressed oil will satisfy your taste for salt. Plus, corn is high in vegetable protein. For expeller-pressed oil and other products you can't find in your supermarket, try the local health food store.
- Frozen cherries, raspberries, or blackberries are a refreshing snack at night. The seeds inside the fruit add fiber, and, although there's not much protein, this fruit is a very complex carbohydrate.

You may be wondering about taking vitamins and food supplements, so let's talk about that.

Vitamins, Minerals, and Food Supplements

Frank Shorter, the United States 1972 gold medalist in the Munich Olympics marathon, was quoted back in the 1980s as having said that he didn't believe in taking vitamins and minerals, but he took them just in case. In my own experience, because of my education, training, and background, companies and individuals have been giving me premium products to try for free for over twenty years. And I have been diligent and fair in trying and evaluating them. I can honestly say that, for the most part, I haven't gained much benefit from them. I'm no pill popper anyway, plus these products are expensive. Like my friend Tom Cremers says, "I'd rather spend my money on wholesome, organic food than on packaged vitamins." I don't want to step on anyone's toes about this issue, however. And my wife and I do take a few daily supplements that we've come to believe in. I'm going to give you some recommendations, but before I do, let me lay a little groundwork.

Vitamins, minerals, and phytonutrients are vital nutrients that exist within the food that the Lord has provided. They are vital for life, though they are needed in smaller amounts. And if you purpose to eat natural, organic, and non-engineered food, you probably don't need to supplement very much. Though they don't produce energy themselves, vitamins and minerals are important because they catalyze and release the energy and other nutrients that are bound in food, helping to control and regulate all the body's cells and organs. But taking pills without eating a healthy diet doesn't do your body much good. I spoke with the owner of a porta-potty company. He told me the main thing he found in his porta-potties was undigested vitamin pills. Avoid the pressed tablet—other sources say about 15 percent of the pressed tablets are absorbed by the body. Your body has been created to recognize what is natural and what is synthetic or engineered. So, if you do choose to take supplements, make sure to research the source and quality of what you're spending your money on. Here's what I recommend:

- Take a whole-food, natural multi-vitamin/mineral each day. No mega doses of anything.
- Take a complete-profile, amino-acid supplement that contains the amino acids of leucine, isoleucine, and valine. Make sure that this capsule-type supplement also contains L-arginine and L-glutamine. These amino acids, which repair tissue, are particularly important for anyone who is doing resistance strength training.
- You may want to take a calcium and magnesium supplement that contains the vitamin B complex.
- It might be a good idea to take an antioxidant supplement. But I'd rather you eat organic fruit and vegetables.
- Taking plant enzymes with your meals may help your digestion. Enzymes are the chemical ingredients in food that speed up the energy release and absorption process within your body.
- I like taking an acidophilus capsule in the morning at breakfast. It provides additional flora and healthy bacteria in the small and large intestines. I've definitely noticed the difference on this one.

I can't honestly recommend you supplement with anything else. Just make sure that whatever you take, you do diligent research. Make sure a supplement is organic, whole, and natural. I know that I've left out a whole lot of information on this topic, but it's way past the scope of this one book. It will probably be addressed in future books that are part of this series on being "Fit to Serve."

Why Organic?

I have to apologize to you. I haven't given you my definition of organically grown food yet. Organic food is fertilized only with only natural fertilizers such as manure, compost, or naturally occurring minerals. They are guaranteed not to have been produced with chemical pesticides and synthetic fertilizers.

Caffeine Consumption

The first thing to consider in consuming coffee, soft drinks, or chocolate is, are you using them for their drug-like effect to get you through your day? If you said yes to this question, the Holy Spirit has probably been trying to have some meaningful discussions with you regarding why you need the extra kicks in the first place.

Caffeine isn't inherently bad for you. It is definitely a brain-to-body stimulant that increases functional performance. Most studies suggest that drinking two to three cups of regular drip coffee (450 mg of caffeine) over the course of your day increases endurance and stamina by up to 20 percent. Moreover, the New England School of Medicine has, on several occasions over the past twenty-five years, published research articles on the effect of drinking coffee and on taking in caffeine in general. All of these articles and studies have consistently stated that, unless a woman is pregnant or someone has fairly serious heart disease, every adult can consume two to three 150 mg caffeinated cups of coffee per day without any issues. I personally drink three cups of organic coffee almost every day without any negative side effects. Having said that, I in no way would encourage anyone to drink coffee or intentionally consume caffeine-containing foods of any kind. If you get negative side effects from coffee or any other caffeinated product, obviously you shouldn't have any.

A great alternative to drinking coffee is green tea. Not only does it have one-third the caffeine, but it's high in minerals and vitamins, especially the antioxidants. I drink it sometimes, and I really like it.

Alcohol

Drinking wine is discussed throughout both the Old and New Testaments. In all of these scriptures, the reader is encouraged to "not be drunk with wine." The Bible does not forbid drinking, but it certainly warns against drinking in front of someone who may have a problem with over-consuming alcohol of any kind. Wine that's produced from real grapes, especially red grapes, does seem to be supported by many authorities as having some positive health benefits. Again, the issue is moderation and frequency.

Drinking beer and hard liquor is another issue. I don't think having a beer here and there is a big deal, but I see a whole lot of people who seem to be affected by the unique combination of barley, hops, and malt. And, of course, the carbonation wreaks havoc on the skeleton, kidneys, and bladder. I don't think drinking hard liquor can be justified on any level. The fermentation process in producing hard liquor or spirits is, in itself, toxic. I have to take a stand and encourage you not to drink any hard liquor. If you are going to drink some wine, choose organic wine to avoid added sulfites or pesticides.

Water

In my opinion, drinking filtered and reverse-osmosis-processed water is the best choice for your body. In purchasing bottled water, make sure that it is pH neutral, neither too acidic nor too alkaline. Also be aware of the plastic container it's bottled in. You may want to consider purchasing a food-grade, stainless-steel drinking container. Just do your due diligence and the Lord will take care of the rest. Try to consume at least two quarts of clean water per day—it's your body's universal lubricant and transport medium. Aside from water bolstering your blood and lymph volumes, its most important function may be its ability to enhance communication from your brain to all seventy-five trillion cells throughout your body. Many authorities believe that chronic dehydration is the greatest cause of disease on the planet. I agree.

Artificial Sweeteners

I'm going to end this chapter by talking about artificial sweeteners. People often look to artificial sweeteners as a way to maintain the amount of food they want to eat. People interested in disease prevention and physical fitness are finally coming to realize you can't fool nature, no matter how much money you spend trying to do so. From saccharine to aspartame to Splenda, they may all end up causing damage to the human body. And for what—so we can eat more food? Instead, eat real food in its natural state and only eat the amount you're really hungry for. Use organic raw sugar, cane sugar, local honey, and pure maple syrup. These natural sweeteners are delicious and, in proper amounts, will contribute to your overall physical fitness. Let's stop with the diet this and the diet that. Realistic nutrition can be summed up by using the sound mind the Lord has given us: whenever possible, make the healthiest choice available and only eat when you're hungry.

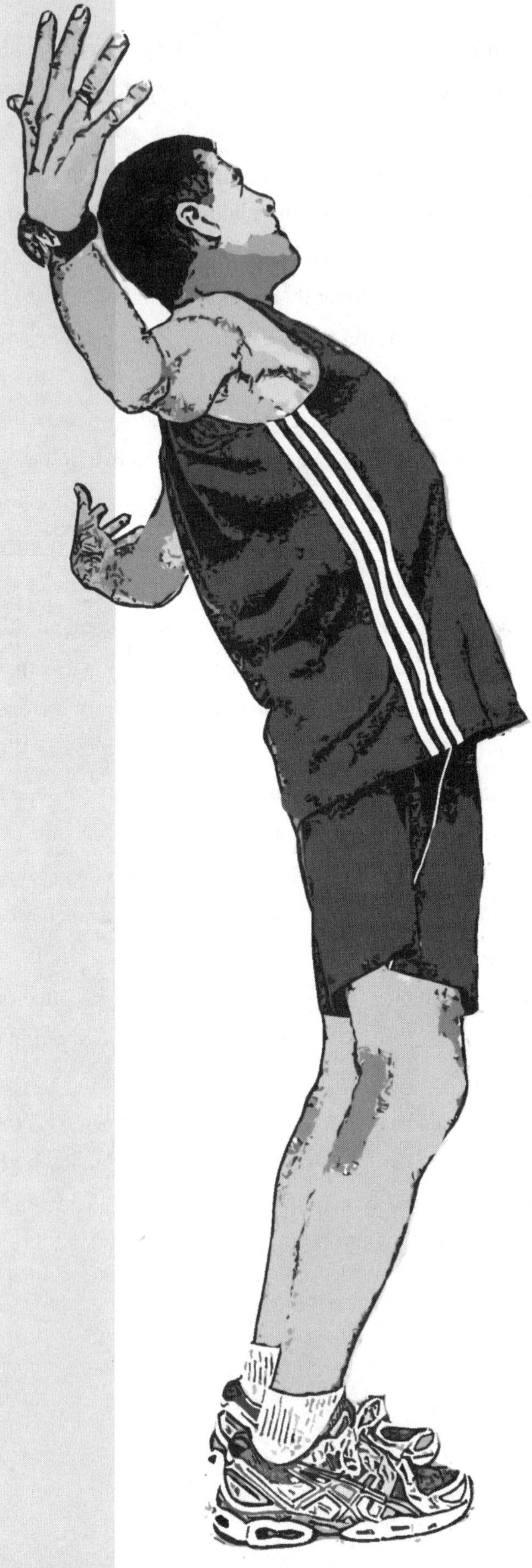

>> *tip:* Eat and Move

Time for a sky reach stretch! Assume an athletic stance. Now look up to the sky and reach as high as you can with both arms. Feel the invigorating stretch of your shoulders, chest, back, and arms. And while you're there, take a deep cleansing breath.

REST AND REGENERATE: GO TO SLEEP

10

Some of my fondest childhood memories involve the bedroom, the bed, and the covers I went to sleep with every night. I love that feeling of getting into a warm bed, covering up with my favorite blanket, and laying my head down on my own special pillow. That feeling of being snug, safe, secure, and at rest is like no other.

Most people I know don't get enough sleep. Parents need to be diligent to provide enough sleep time for their children. I commonly meet school-aged children who are chronically sleep-deprived and adults that have even more severe sleep deprivation.

J. Allan Holson, director of the Laboratory of Neurophysiology at Harvard, says that quality dream sleep is critical in the brain development of children. But adults need sleep too. It is a common misconception that the older you are the less sleep you need. I see this behavior in adults who are forty to seventy years old all the time. They go to sleep by ten and get up at four as a matter of course. Six or fewer hours of sleep each night is not enough for maximum physical fitness. For the most part, every human needs seven to nine hours of peaceful sleep every night.

"For the most part, every human needs seven to nine hours of peaceful sleep every night."

Consistent, high quality sleep allows our bodies and our minds to restore and repair after all the circumstances that occurred during the day.

Jesus knew the importance of sleep. The Bible shows Jesus sleeping like a baby, even in the middle of a violent storm. Now, that's sleeping soundly. In Psalm 4:8, King David writes, "I will lie down in peace and sleep, for you alone, O Lord, will keep me safe." And in Psalm 127:2, he says, "It is useless for you to work so hard from early morning until late at night, anxiously working for food to eat; for God gives rest to his loved ones."

Not too many years ago, people used to talk about trying to get ahead and living the good life as being "caught up in the rat race." I haven't heard that expression in quite a while, but it's more applicable than ever. People are in a frantic race to work harder and harder to buy more and more. Have you noticed people don't park their automobiles in their garages anymore? That's because their garages are packed with stuff—stuff they've worked their fingers to the bone for, stuff they never use. I know people who keep adding more metal buildings to their property so they can store more boats, motorcycles, and other toys.

In Ecclesiastes, King Solomon, one of the richest men who ever lived, says that the poor man had as much joy as he had. Joy is taking time to appreciate the life and love that we have. In his book *The Seven Pillars of Health,* Dr. Don Colbert gives five reasons why sleep and rest are so important for your physical fitness.*

1. *Sleep regulates the release of important hormones.* When you sleep, growth hormone is secreted. This causes children to grow, and it regulates muscle mass and helps control fat in adults. When you don't sleep enough, this hormone's function is disrupted. Perhaps lack of sleep is partially to blame for the fact that two-thirds of Americans are overweight or obese. Leptin, another hormone, is secreted during sleep and directly influences appetite and weight control. It tells the body when it is "full." A person who doesn't have enough of this regulating hormone often has a runaway appetite.
2. *Sleep slows the aging process.* The term "beauty rest" is literally true. Sleep slows the aging process, and some say it is one of the most important "secrets" for averting wrinkles. How well a person sleeps is one of the most important predictors of how long that person will live.
3. *Sleep boosts the immune system.* People who sleep nine hours a night instead of seven hours have greater than normal "natural killer cell" activity. Natural killer cells destroy viruses, bacteria, and cancer.
4. *Sleep improves brain function.* One study shows that even short-term sleep deprivation may decrease brain activity related to alertness and cognitive performance.
5. *Sleep reduces cortisol levels.* Excessive stress raises cortisol levels, which disrupt neurotransmitter balance in the brain, causing you to be more irritable and prone to depression, anxiety, and insomnia. High cortisol levels are associated with many diseases, but the cure is as close as your pillow. Sufficient sleep helps to reduce cortisol levels.

Create Your Haven of Rest

Ever since I was a young boy I've known in my heart the importance of creating an environment for getting a great night's sleep. Both the bed and the bedroom have to be enhanced for you to have rest and regeneration.

* Excerpt taken from Don Colbert, MD, *The Seven Pillars of Health* (Lake Mary: Siloam, 2007), 38–39.

The Bedroom

The bedroom, or at least the bed area, should be soft, warm, and comfortable in terms of décor, lighting, and mood. It should be quiet, private, and well ventilated. You should feel safe and secure when you slip into bed. Try to have it as dark as possible. You want your conscious and subconscious mind to perceive that it is absolutely time to go to sleep. The moment you shut the lights off, your soul should say, "Yes!"

By the way, creating total darkness during sleep hours is critical for people who have to work at night. The Lord created humans to be diurnal (day) creatures. We're supposed to be awake during the day and asleep during the night. If you're forced to work nights, you're going to have to go to great lengths to create an environment where your day becomes your night and your night becomes your day. Otherwise, all of the sleep deprivation will be compounded even more. This means no phone calls, sirens, kids yelling, or someone knocking on the door. Ensuring this environment is not selfish. If you get the right amount of sleep, you'll be a better Christian, a better husband or wife, a better parent, a better friend, and a better employee or business owner.

The Bed

Now let's talk about the bed itself. The bed is the one piece of furniture where you should spare no expense. At the writing of this book, my youngest daughter, Krista, is preparing to marry. She and her fiancé are both young missionaries, so money is a real issue. They were recently shopping for their bed and came to the point of making their choice and purchase. It was more than they wanted to spend, so Krista called Rebecca to talk about it. Rebecca was quick to tell her that the extra investment will pay them back thousands of times in the quality of their lives and their walk with the Lord.

Choose a bed that's just right for you. It doesn't have to be the most expensive one, but it has to be the best one for you. My wife is constantly tweaking the comfort of our bed. She experiments with mattress pads, memory foam, and even the thread count of our sheets and pillowcases. I love her for it, and I love our bed.

Your Bedtime Routine

All the systems of your mind and body are subject to one of life's greatest secrets: you become what you think about. So, if you want to get a good night's sleep, you have to plan for it by creating a routine of habits that lead up to it. I actually start thinking about going to bed by mid-afternoon. Rebecca and I usually go for an aerobic fitness walk right before we sit down in our matching, swivel rocking chairs. Then we begin decompressing from our day. We get a delicious beverage in our favorite porcelain cups and start talking about everything—our children, our friends, what we accomplished that day, and what the Lord is doing in our lives. Next, we prepare a simple but nutritious and delicious dinner. After that, we enjoy soft, uplifting music and pleasant conversation. As darkness falls on the day, we retire to the bedroom. We may have a light snack and watch a little television. Then comes lights out and we say to one another, "Ahhh.... Good night, honey. I love you." No distress, no anxiety, just peace and tranquility.

>> *tip:* **Eat and Move**

Have a small bowl of crispy organic blue corn chips. These chips are an ancient tradition of the Hopi and Zuni Indian tribes. They'll hit the spot and get ya going!

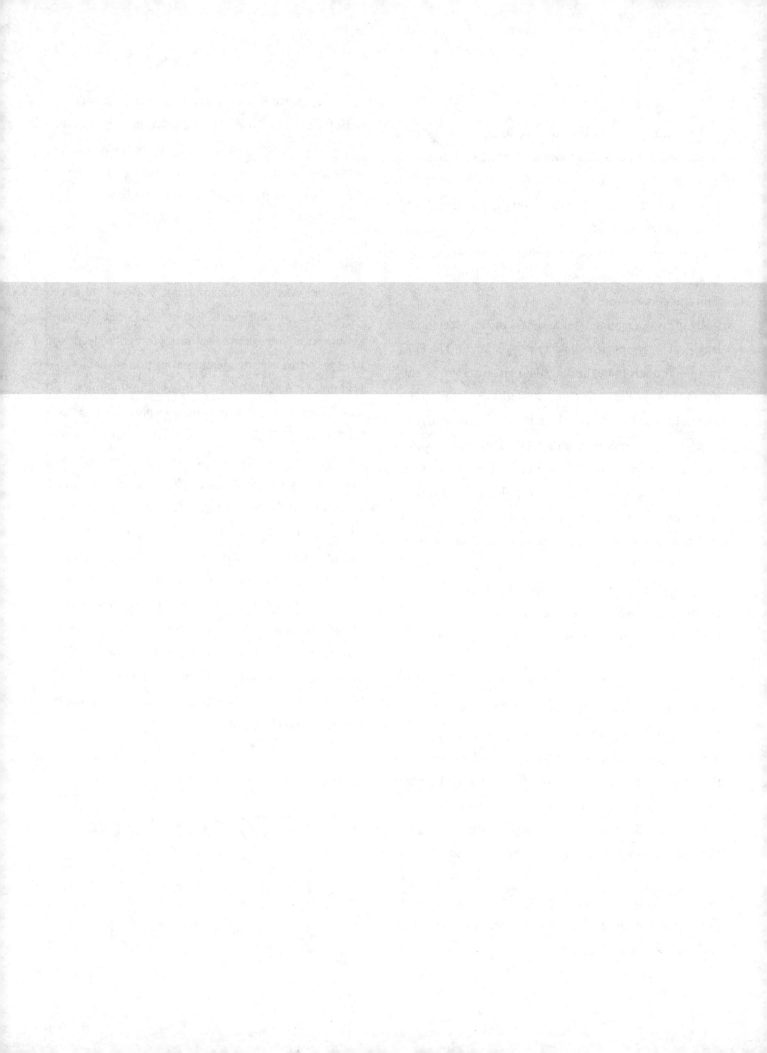

Part Three: **The Action Plan**

Now we come to the fun part. I say that because it's the *doing* of fitness that has given me so much pleasure and joy over the years.

The real key to improving your physical fitness lies in developing and adopting an action plan. So, in this next part, I offer you a system so that you will achieve positive, effective, and permanent change in your life. Who knows? Maybe you too will become an ambassador of physical fitness.

CARDIOVASCULAR/RESPIRATORY EXERCISE

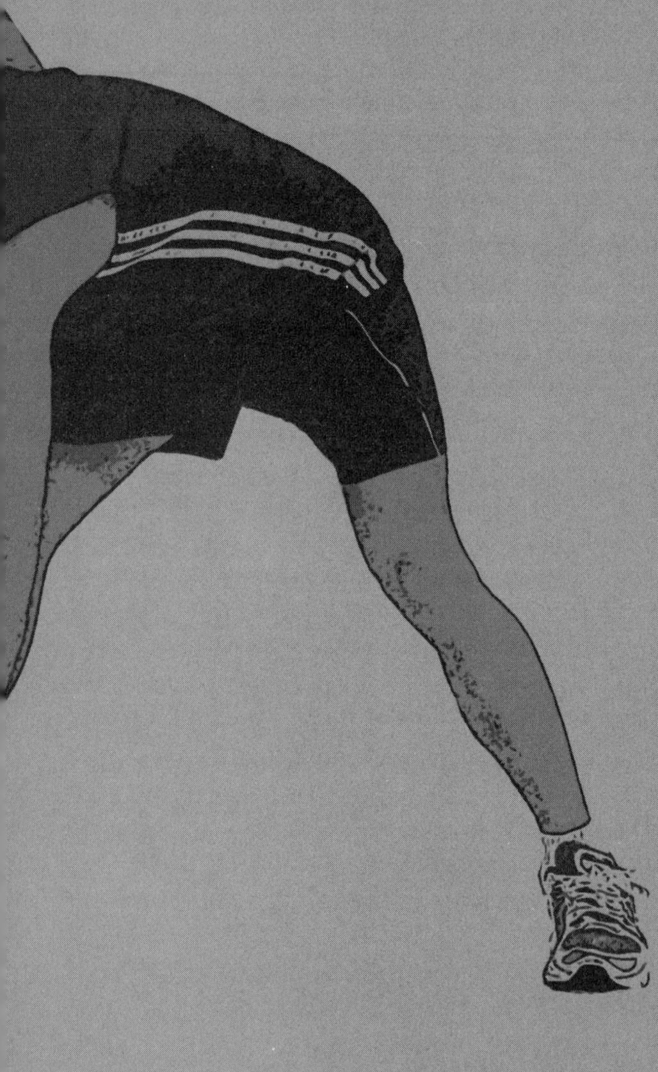

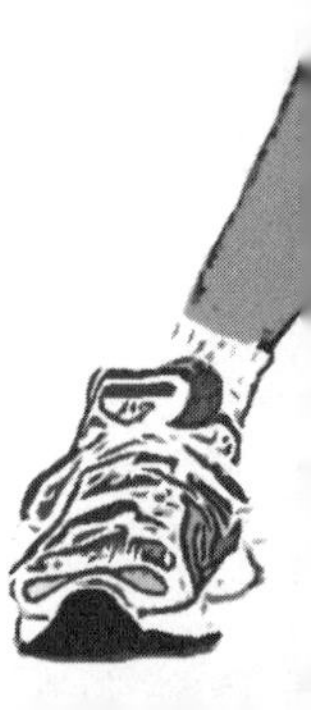

11

Cardiovascular/Respiratory exercise conditions your heart, circulatory pathways, and lungs. In terms of body composition, cardiovascular training improves the body's ability to release and burn fat as a primary source of fuel, provided that the training follows the appropriate level of intensity. Glucose and stored body fat supply the primary fuel for this type of exercise. That's why most people who exercise prefer to do aerobics. *Aerobic* means "with oxygen." They want to decrease their body fat, so they think aerobic exercise is best.

Their thinking is partially correct. They are burning fat, but remember, the primary benefit of aerobics is conditioning the heart and lungs and clearing the vascular pathways. So, enthusiasts often spend too much time in their aerobic conditioning, exercising at a high level of intensity that burns sugar and protein along with fat. The result is the breakdown and decrease of their lean body mass. They become skinny, flabby people or bags of bones. Yes, they're thin, but they don't look healthy. Instead, they look drawn and emaciated, dried up and old. This type of exercise is the one that most often becomes a compulsive disorder and a negative addiction.

It happened to me in the mid- to late-seventies. I had decided to try out for the U.S. Olympic Team in marathon running for the 1980 Summer Games in Moscow, Russia. I began stepping up my running distance gradually from five miles per day, six days a week, to twenty-five miles per day, six days per week. I had to run at least two to three times a day to get that 150 miles a week logged in.

At Christmas I was home from college. It was a severely cold winter in Green Bay, Wisconsin. Daytime temperatures were well below zero, but I had to get my runs in, no matter what. I coated my face with Vaseline, watched icicles

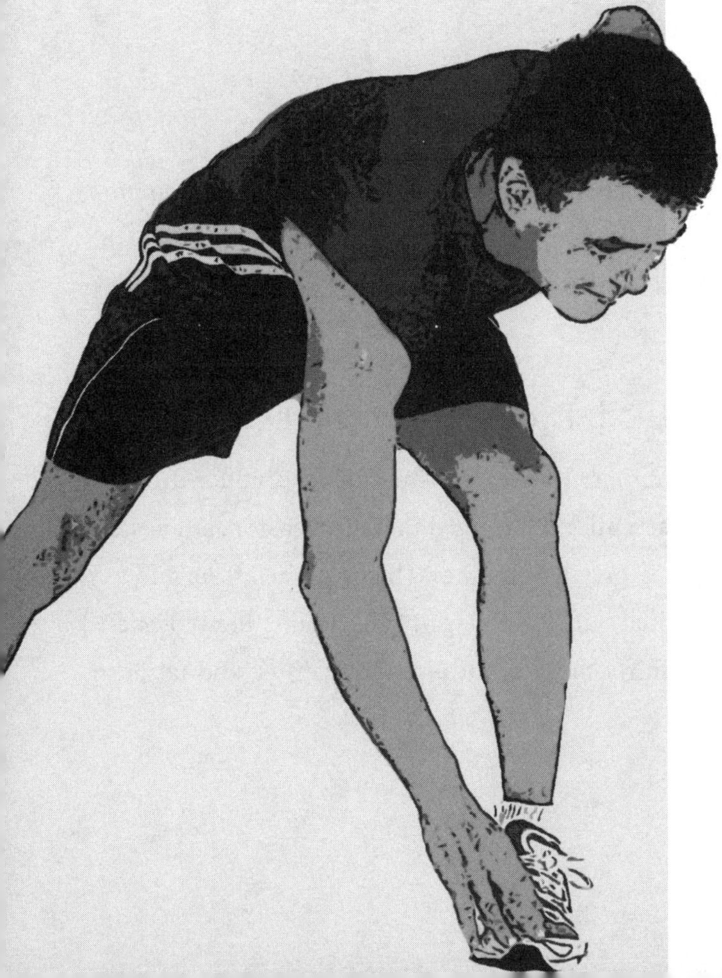

form on my mustache, and even resorted to wearing bread bags over my gloves to protect myself from the bitter cold. Sweat froze inside the bag. Large chunks of frozen sweat fell off my hat. One day, as I was getting ready to walk out the door to begin my run, my mother confronted me, standing with her hands on her hips. "Timothy, running is your god! You're crazy to go out in this cold."

I shrugged her off, and took the run anyway. But eight months later, the reality of her words came crashing down on my head. I was in graduate school in Huntsville, Texas. It was the middle of August, and I was out for my afternoon run. About halfway into that run I felt a tug on the back of my left thigh. I stopped and stretched a bit before finishing the run. The next morning, I got up and went out for my morning run. After about a mile, the muscles in the backs of both my thighs locked down tight. Suddenly I could barely walk, much less run. I had to hitchhike back to my apartment. As soon as I got there, the pain set in—a burning, prickly pain. I also had numbness in my hands and feet.

It scared me to death and put me in a wheelchair. As it turned out, the U.S. Olympic team never went to Moscow because President Carter declared a boycott. But I was unable to run for eight years, and even had to drop out of college.

In the end, after countless doctors and numerous tests, I was diagnosed with an overuse injury. I had damaged, and my body had ingested, the protective sheaths that encapsulated the major nerves of the muscles in the back of my thighs (the hamstrings).

Running had indeed become my god, and the price of my sin was despair, pain, and tissue destruction. The huge silver lining to this story, however, is that it brought me to repentance. I accepted Jesus as my Lord and Savior. It also brought me to Rebecca, the woman who became my bride and my lifelong partner now of twenty-eight years.

I found I could worship and honor God with my experience. I also learned that too much of a good thing can become a bad thing. My aerobic conditioning was extremely out of balance with the other components of my physical fitness.

Back in the late seventies, Dr. Kenneth Cooper of the Aerobics Research Center in Dallas, Texas, gave the essential principles for effective aerobic conditioning. His study showed that to condition the cardiovascular/respiratory system, you had to exercise only 20 to 30 minutes, three to four times a week, at an intensity of 60 to 85 percent of your maximum heart rate. For the most part, his findings have withstood the test of time and are still valid today. Can you safely exercise aerobically more than thirty minutes, four days a week? Yes, but not too much. Anything past sixty minutes, six days per week, and you're asking for problems. Let's go over these principles.

Aerobic Conditioning Principles

Frequency: Three to Six Days per Week

Anything under three days a week, and you won't develop and maintain cardiovascular and respiratory health. Anything over six days and you're violating the Sabbath day principle of taking time for rest, recovery, and growth.

Duration: Twenty to Sixty Minutes

A number of government studies conducted in the early seventies determined that the ideal for aerobic exercise was forty-five minutes. This gives you fifteen minutes for initial burning of sugar, kick-starting thermogenesis, then thirty minutes for arterial cleansing and fat burning.

Intensity: 50 to 90 Percent of Predicted Maximum Heart Rate

Even though you can physically justify exercising aerobically at an intensity between 70 and 90 percent of your predicted maximum heart rate, I don't recommend it. Again, once you pass 75 percent maximum intensity, your body goes from burning fat to consuming lean body mass, as well as necessary hormones. I want you to decrease your body fat while increasing your lean body mass. The key is to keep your exercise intensity right at 70 percent.

Calculating Exercise Heart Rate Intensity

The American College of Sports Medicine Method

To get your predicted maximum heart rate, subtract your age from 220 (a newborn baby's heart rate). Then, multiply your predicted maximum heart rate by the desired exercise intensity. See figure 11.1 for an example.

FIGURE 11.1 CALCULATE HEART RATE

220 (newborn heart rate) – 54 (my age now)
= 166

166 x 70% or 0.7 (percent exercise intensity)
= 116

Heart beats per minute exercise intensity
= 116

Note: Most people consider this method overly conservative. The next method is one that many endurance athletes prefer.

The Maffleton Method

Subtract your age from 180, which gives you approximately an aerobic exercise intensity 75 percent of your maximum heart rate. Here's an example:

180
– 54
= 126 Beats per minute

Subtract five points if you're just getting started.

Add five points if you're a competitive endurance athlete.

Monitoring Your Heart Rate

There are several ways you can check your heart rate in order to monitor your intensity: Wear a heart rate monitor. It'll cost about $100 for a good one. If you don't have a heart rate monitor, evaluate manually by putting your fingertips lightly on the carotid artery at the base of your neck.

Take your pulse on the inside of your wrist. Make sure to use four fingers, not your thumb, to feel for your pulse because your thumb has its own beat.

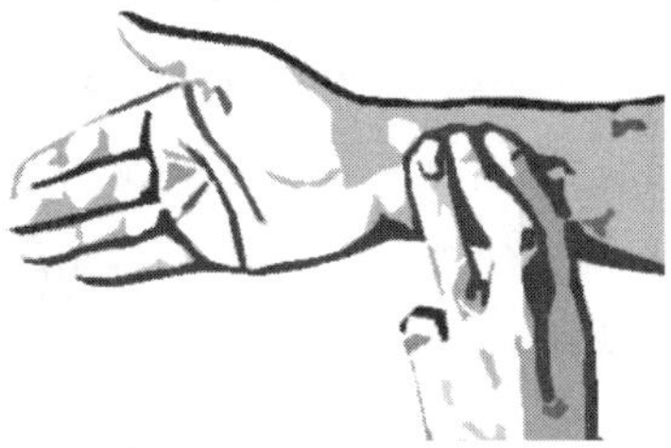

FIGURE 11.2 TAKE YOUR PULSE AT THE WRIST

Count the number of beats for ten seconds and multiply by six to get a sixty second pulse rate. It's okay if your exercise heart rate is five beats over or under the heart rate you want—that's close enough.

Aerobic Exercise Activities

Power Walking

Fitness walking, or power walking, as I like to call it, is the best overall aerobic exercise. You can walk anywhere. You don't need a fitness membership or special clothing. All you need is a good pair of shoes. Here are the mechanics.

1. Initiate a heel strike at the front of your heel on the bottom of your shoe. Roll the foot forward and push off the back of the ball of your foot.

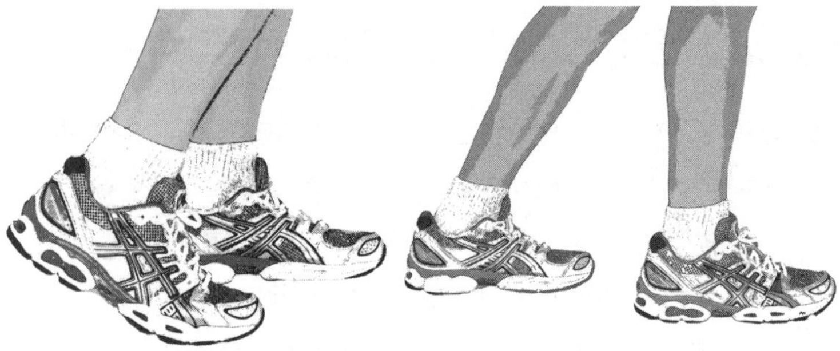

FIGURE 11.3 POWER WALKING

2. Keep your knees bent at least two inches. This knee bend will cushion the foot force and will help you land your foot straight under your hips.
3. As you walk, keep your feet hip-width apart, like you're walking on separate train tracks. This will keep your hip, knee, and foot in a direct line of push and pull, and will decrease the torque on your back, knees, and ankles.
4. Keep a slight bend in your elbow and let your hands swing naturally as you walk.
5. Walk briskly at a speed just under a slow jog. Adjust this speed according to your desired heart rate.

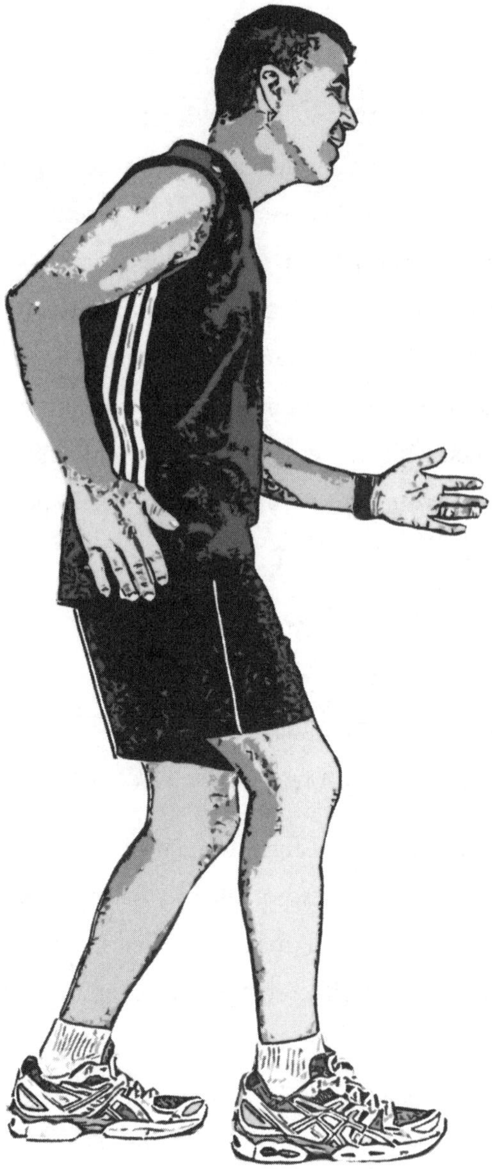

FIGURE 11.4 POWER WALKING: PUTTING THE MECHANICS TOGETHER

"Fitness walking, or power walking, as I like to call it, is the best overall aerobic exercise. You can walk anywhere."

Light Jogging

Light jogging is the next speed up from power walking. But be careful. I really don't recommend running at an intensity that raises your heartbeat more than 75 percent of your predicted maximum heart rate. That's when your body begins to consume lean body mass. So, if you're going to distance run, make sure you monitor your heart rate and keep it at or below 75 percent of your predicted maximum heart rate.

Your mechanics should be the same as the power walk, with the exception of your foot strike initiation. Your jogging foot strike should initiate at the back of the ball of your foot and end with the front of your heel coming down lightly. This is referred to as the mid-foot strike.

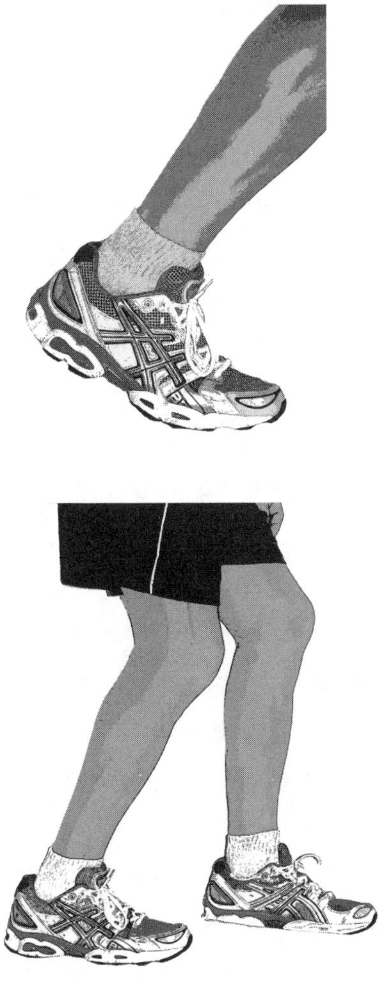

Figure 11.5 Foot strike in jogging

Outdoor Cycling

Outdoor cycling is fun and an excellent aerobic exercise. It's also easier on your joints than jogging because the bike unloads the downward foot strike force. Of course, you will have to compensate by increasing your speed. You don't have to have an expensive or fancy bike, just one in good working order. Here are some considerations.

1. Please wear a helmet. Statistics show that head injuries are the number-one injury in recreational cycling.
2. Wear shoes to provide support and protect your feet. Sandals are inappropriate for biking.
3. Anchor the ball of your foot on the center of the bike pedal.
4. Your knee should have a slight bend in it at the bottom of your stroke.

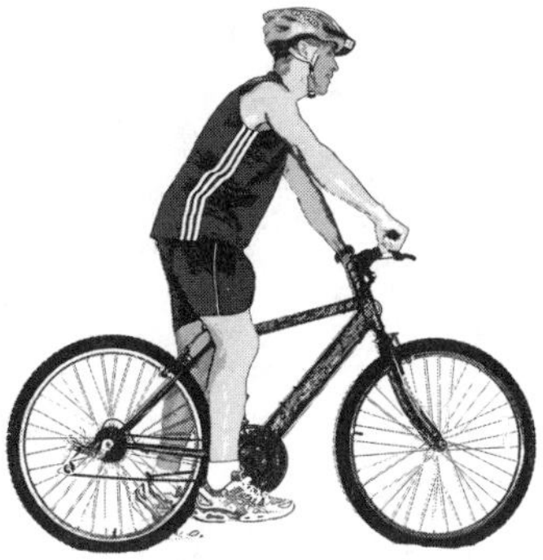

Figure 11.6 Wear a helmet and keep a slight bend in the knee

5. Handlebar heights
   - Recreational—handlebars are higher than the seat
   - Triathlete—handlebars are even with the seat
   - Professional cyclist—handlebars are below the seat
6. Tire pressure: keep the tires at the recommended psi. Avoid over- or underinflation.

Open Water and Lap Swimming

Swimming is awesome aerobic exercise. Your skeletal mass actually floats inside your body when you're submerged in water, thus your joints are unloaded. Swimming is a whole-body exercise movement, no matter which stroke you are using, so you burn a lot of energy. Swimming is considered a superior cardiovascular/respiratory exercise because the heart does not have to overcome the gravity effect. When your body is horizontal in water, the heart receives a maximum stroke volume of blood per heartbeat. Because of this, your swimming heart rate is about ten beats per minute less than an equivalent upright aerobic activity.

Many public swimming pools offer affordable lessons if you need instruction or a tune-up for your swim strokes. Maintaining rhythm and intensity is key and will leave you feeling invigorated.

FIGURE 11.7 SELECT A STROKE OR COMBINATION OF STROKES

Please be careful when swimming in open waters. Always swim with a buddy, and be mindful of weather and shoreline conditions. Also be aware of chlorine levels in swimming pools. Goggles will protect your eyes, a cap will protect your hair, and a good soapy shower afterward will protect your skin.

Indoor Aerobic Machines

Treadmills

I believe that walking on a natural surface is superior to walking on a treadmill. Your brain definitely knows what's natural. However, sometimes you may have to use a treadmill because of weather conditions (rain, heat, cold, etc.). The advantage of a treadmill over natural walking is that it makes you maintain a set pace and a steady heart-rate intensity. If you use a treadmill, I prefer you use the "manual mode" so that you can keep your heart rate at that fat burning intensity.

Stationary Bicycles

I prefer a sit-back recumbent bike over an upright bike because it's easier on the back, knees, ankles, and feet. You can also brace your back on a recumbent bike. The same mechanics apply to indoor cycles as to regular outdoor bicycles, except you don't need a helmet indoors (unless you want to get a few laughs, of course).

Elliptical Trainers

These devices have really become mainstream and have withstood the test of time. The movement is horizontally oval and unloads vertical force that comes up from the foot in walking, running, and cycling. It's not a natural movement, however, so you'll have to closely monitor your exercise heart rate.

Stair-climbers/Steppers

These machines are great at simulating the natural climbing of stairs. I get a kick out of people who use these machines at their fitness clubs only to take escalators and elevators when they're in buildings, stores, and airports. The joint angles required in a stepping motion are great for conditioning your legs and hips. But once again, because you're compounding the effects of gravity in stepping up, you'll have to monitor your heart rate.

Throughout this chapter, I've emphasized that you not exceed 75 percent of your predicted maximum heart rate. This doesn't mean that I don't want you to get your heart rate high. In the next chapter, I'm going to show you how exercises with short bursts of maximum intensity will release productive hormones, condition your total body, and burn only sugar. Just remember that, to get the best aerobic conditioning, we want to get your heart rate up and keep it at a steady intensity.

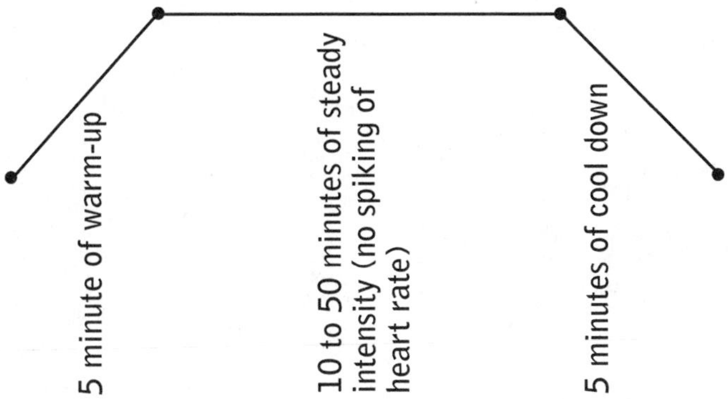

FIGURE 11.8 STEADY HEART RATE

>> *tip:* Eat and Move

Do a set of body weight squats—twenty repetitions. Make sure to keep your head up and your lower back slightly arched as you perform the movements. Try to get as deep as you can. These are great for you hips, thighs, abdomen, and lower back.

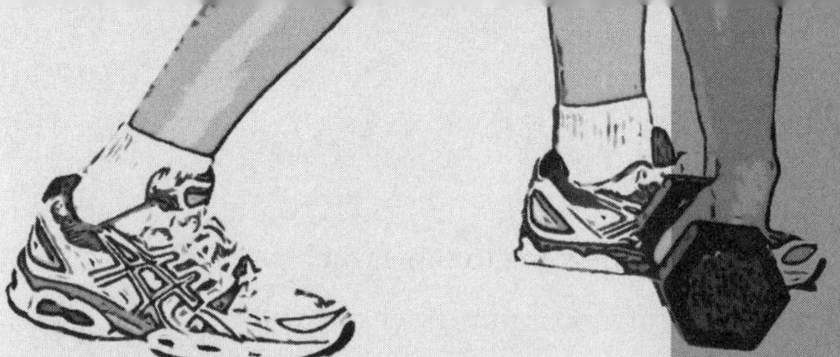

MUSCULAR/SKELETAL STRENGTH DEVELOPMENT

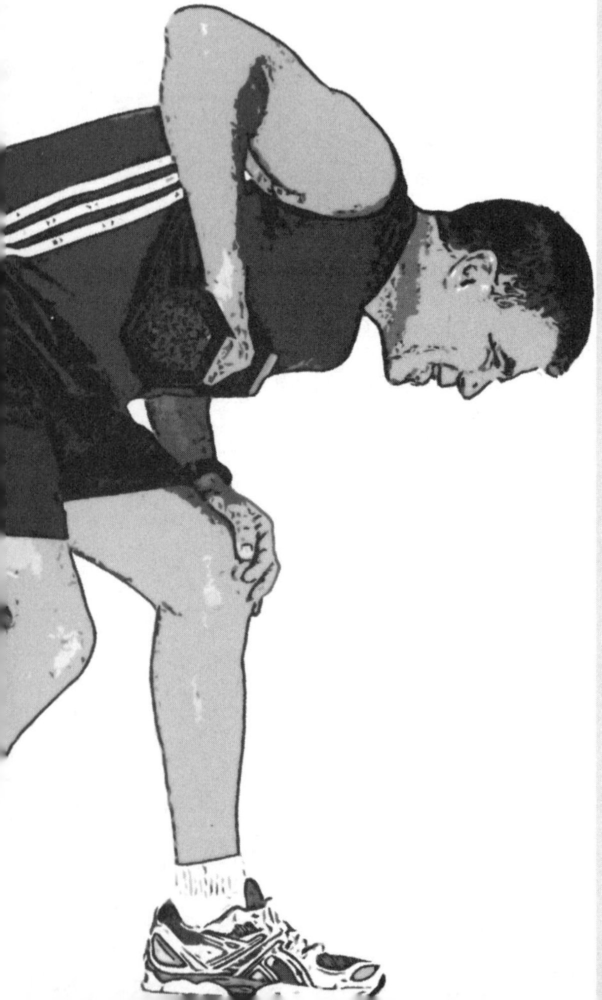

12

When were you in your glory days? When were you at your best and in your prime? You probably came up with a time and date immediately, but it was a trick question. I want your answer to be that you're in your glory days right now! The Lord Almighty is a God of process. He wants us to develop and become more and more like his Son Jesus over time. I believe that we should be spiritually, mentally, emotionally, and, in many ways, physically at our best in the now.

"I believe that we should be spiritually, mentally, emotionally, and, in many ways, physically at our best in the now."

I think it's very interesting that in Psalm 92:10, King David proclaims that God has made him as strong as a wild bull. Have you ever taken the time to really look at a prize bull? It embodies fierceness and immensity. Its strength and raw power is almost immeasurable. I doubt it would back down from anything in nature.

In my own life, I was physically the strongest that I ever was in 1973 and 1974. At the time, I was working as a bridge and building carpenter for the Chicago and Northwestern Railroad in northeast Wisconsin. We worked with classic railroad ties, each one weighing three hundred pounds. One workday, I and another fellow had to unload a train stacked with a few hundred of these ties. We made short order of that load.

I was so physically strong at that time in my life that I could pick up the back end of an automobile by myself. The reason I was so strong was that I was regularly lifting and straining against heavy things.

Strength development is one of the most neglected components of physical fitness, especially by women and middle-aged men. But now, strength training is coming into fashion as people discover its incredible benefits. I've already defined muscular/skeletal strength as the ability to exert force. There are a number of components of strength that I want you to be aware of.

Components of Strength

Absolute Strength

Absolute strength is the maximum amount of force that you can exert against something with conscious thought for one repetition.

Limit Strength

Limit strength is the maximum amount of force that you can exert against something with reflexive, unconscious thought. An example of this is the grandma who picks up an automobile to free her trapped grandchild.

Stamina

Muscular stamina is the ability to maintain your strength over an extended period of time. An example of this would be an American football player who is as strong in the fourth quarter of play as he was in the first quarter.

Power

Power is probably the most day-to-day and real-life application of strength. Power is the ability to exert maximum force against something in the fastest possible time. An example of this would be picking up a bag of dry cement and in one motion hoisting it up onto the back of a pickup truck. Power is a dynamic strength. When a baseball player swings a bat, he is expressing power.

Endurance

Muscular endurance is the ability to continue contracting your muscles at a low level of force for an extended period of time without needing to stop and rest.

The latest findings from exercise scientists tell us that when we do strength training for an endurance sport, such as cycling, our overall performance also improves. The stronger a muscle becomes, the less exertion is needed to perform. This concept is called "economy of movement."

Functional Strength

The Lord wants you and me to be strong for his purposes, not our purposes, and certainly not for vain attempts to be the "body beautiful." No, I believe the Lord wants us functionally strong to carry out the Great Commission, telling others about Jesus.

Functional strength is developed by performing whole-body directional movements that integrate your body. The adage we use is "train movements, not muscles." When you train your body through movements, you will of course be conditioning your muscles. It would be impossible not to. However, the emphasis is on performance, not appearance.

The best way to be strong, muscular, lean, and tight is through proper strength training. That means the process of recruiting more and more of your nerves and muscle mass in a given exercise. More about this later.

Benefits of Strength

Skeletal Strength and Durability

Bones, joints, and connective tissues don't contract, but they do store energy, flex, twist, bend, and exert force. As you strength train and load force onto your body, it responds by increasing the bone mineral density and collagen content of all the hard tissues. It's like going from a forty-pound bow to a sixty-pound bow. The heavier the bow, the farther and faster an arrow will travel. This is what happens to your skeleton when you strength train and condition. The increase in bone mineral density and collagen content also increases your ability to bend and not break, like if you are ever in an accident of some kind.

Body Fat Reduction

Developing and improving the various facets of your strength will shape and tone your muscles and help you perform tasks with greater ease. It's also the best way to decrease your body fat.

About ten years ago I read a book written by Covert Bailey, a well-known exercise physiologist. He said the reason heavy resistance training was better at reducing body fat than aerobic conditioning was that weight training utilized stored sugar from within the muscles (my paraphrase). Depleting the muscles of their sugar forces the brain to signal for stored body fat to be sent to the muscles for immediate fuel. This refueling process increases the thermogenic response a whopping two and a half times that of aerobic conditioning. The leanest and best-looking bodies belong to those people who balance their aerobic conditioning with their anaerobic resistance exercise through weight training and sprints.

Let's look again at a modified weekly exercise schedule (figure 12.1) with this concept in mind.

Anabolic Protein Synthesis

The reason that anaerobic resistance exercise builds lean body mass is that when the structural integrity of muscle and bone is broken down, your brain goes immediately into restoring and repairing that tissue through a production or *synthesis* that results in the building up (that is, *anabolic*) of muscle and bone (*protein*).

What's absolutely amazing is that the Lord created your body with the intelligence to recognize that, if it doesn't compensate for the physical stress you're imposing upon

Day of the Week	Morning Workout	Afternoon Workout
Monday	Strength workout	Aerobic workout
Tuesday	Sprint workout	Aerobic workout
Wednesday	Strength workout	Aerobic workout
Thursday	Sprint workout	Aerobic workout
Friday	Strength workout	Aerobic workout
Saturday	Sprint workout	Aerobic workout
Sunday	The Lord's day is for fellowship, rest, and growth	

FIGURE 12.1 WEEKLY EXERCISE SCHEDULE MODEL—MODIFIED TO INCLUDE RUNNING, SWIMMING, AND CYCLING SPRINTS

it by increasing its ability to withstand this stress, it would become injured, dysfunctional, or dead.

The reason that athletes who do only aerobic conditioning have low muscularity is that they never break muscle down so that it has the opportunity to rebuild. They don't allow it to repair and grow. To me, this is unhealthy. It's not physical fitness.

Training Frequency

Earlier I identified most of the essentials for muscular strength development. Let's review and look a little deeper at training frequency.

Two Days per Week

The minimum number of days that you can strength train and sustain a benefit is twice a week. Your workouts must be within four days or ninety-six hours of the previous workout.

Three Days per Week

This is the best schedule for the beginning strength trainer because it allows forty-eight hours of recovery and growth, and balances the necessary duration and the number of different exercises you need to do.

Four-Day Split Routine

In my opinion, this is the best possible system for those who aren't beginners. It gives you 25 percent more volume of exercise over the three-day schedule, yet allows you to invest training time in the other necessary components of physical fitness.

Five- and Six-Day Splits

Strength training five or six days per week is primarily for the person that wants to build up the size of his or her muscles. The downside of bodybuilding is that time is being taken away from the other physical fitness components. Bodybuilders may have a high level of strength, but this strength is developed specifically for the movement they perform to build their enlarged muscles. Actually, bodybuilders are fairly weak in relation to their body weight. Their bodies are not functionally fit to carry out everyday activities.

Workout Duration

Dr. Barry Sears, in his book *Enter the Zone,* says, if a person strains in a workout with movements lasting much past forty-five to sixty minutes, the brain and body perceive tissue trauma and respond by dumping cortisol into the bloodstream.*

Cortisol is a great hormone when you're in a crisis situation, like running for your life. But if you regularly cause the production and release of cortisol, it breaks down your lean body mass's ability to recover, repair, and grow before your next workout. This is when injuries occur and the process of "over-training" begins.

So, keep all of your workouts under an hour. It takes about two to three hours for cortisol to calm down in the body before you can go again. This is one reason I recommend morning and afternoon workouts.

Workout Basics

Upper Body Workouts

You need to perform at least six to eight different exercises for at least three sets each to comprehensively train your upper body. Your upper body is the back, chest, shoulders, and arms. This is also the order to train the upper body. It should take approximately forty-five minutes.

* Barry Sears, *Enter the Zone* (New York: Regan Books, 1997).

Lower Body Workouts

Training your lower body calls for exercising your hips, core, and legs. The core of your body includes from just below your belly button up to your bottom rib, 360 degrees around your middle. Your core is interconnected with twenty-nine different muscle groups. So, when you condition your abdominals, you're also conditioning your back, and vice versa. Of course, everything in your body is interrelated and interconnected.

Your lower body will also require at least six to eight different exercises whenever you are targeting this area. You will need to allow for more recovery time between your sets because the lower body involves much larger muscle groups. Thus, lower body workouts will require the full sixty minutes. In fact, you'll often find yourself running out of time. Do the best you can in sixty minutes. Don't go over.

Whole Body Strength Workouts

Your weekly schedule may demand you do both upper and lower body workouts at one time. You'll have to push to do it in sixty minutes, but it can be done. Just know that you'll probably have to leave some exercises for your next workout. That's okay. Exercise is not an exact science. And like we say often, the most important things are to show up and work hard!

Training Intensities

Training intensity means how hard you're pushing yourself and straining. Intensity requires going to the point of momentary muscular failure, where you have to stop and rest. The other part of intensity is how many repetitions you can do at a given load or weight. This information on repetitions, sets, and speed of movement comes from Mel Cunningham Siff's definitive work, *Supertraining.**

To Increase Absolute Strength

To get strong, you're going to have to lift heavy weights. I will explain a little later how to lift heavy weights. Obviously, you can't start with extreme loads without getting hurt. So, a methodology will be provided.

"To get strong, you're going to have to lift weights."

Repetitions per Exercise

A standard set is one to eight repetitions. Most strength development experts recommend performing four to six repetitions to the point of momentary failure.

Sets per Exercise

The usual number of sets is four to seven. Most strength coaches will have you move onto another exercise after five sets. However, you may perform an additional sixth or seventh set if you're performing an extremely large movement that is using a high number of muscle groups. The barbell squat is an example: it sometimes takes the full seven sets for a lifter to get to the highest weight.

Speed of Movement

If your goal is to get stronger rather than making your muscles look bigger, then the amount of weight you lift is most important. Your speed of movement should be at a "one-to-one count." For example, while doing a biceps curl, raise the weight up by flexing at the elbow for a "one thousand one" count. That raising and lowering of the weight makes up one repetition.

* Mel Cunningham Siff, *Supertraining* (Denver: The Supertraining Institute, 2003).

Muscular Stamina

Stamina—the ability to sustain a high level of strength over an extended period of time—is developed the same way as absolute strength, with the exception of the number of repetitions. For stamina, do six to eight repetitions instead of four to six. The higher the repetitions, the greater the endurance of the muscle group.

Muscular-Skeletal Power

Power is the ability to move weight fast. So, if you want to develop power in your movements, you have to perform them fast, just like you would in real life. Power development is basically identical to strength development, except it's done at a faster speed.

Let's look at the biceps curl again. To develop strength you performed the movement at a one-to-one count, up and then back down. To develop power in this same movement, you would perform at a 0.5-to-1.0 count. That would mean raising the weight in a half-second, but lowering and controlling it back down *still at one-second speed.* Going back down slower avoids damaging the muscles, nerves, and joints. Another difference between strength and power development is limiting the total number of sets at three to five, instead of four to seven.

Muscular Endurance

To develop bodily and muscular endurance—that is, continuing to contract your muscles at a lower resistance but for an extended period of time—the following principles will apply.

Repetitions per Exercise

The number of repetitions for developing endurance is fifteen to sixty. Most endurance coaches will have you do between twenty-five and forty repetitions. Once the resistance is low enough that you can continue performing past forty repetitions, it's considered too light and the benefit will be minimal.

Sets per Exercise

Resistance in endurance development is so low that the risk of injury is also low. And because you won't use your total nerve and muscle mass to overcome a resistance, performing higher numbers of sets is unnecessary. So, the number of sets is two to four. I'd recommend no more than three.

Speed of Movement

To understand the speed of movement, think of things you do over and over again at a low resistance. Walking is a good example. When you walk somewhere, even at a brisk pace, your movements aren't explosive. They're even and steady. We've found that the best speed of exercise movements to develop muscular endurance is slightly slower than the speed to develop strength. Strength is best developed at a one-to-one count in raising and lowering the weight. For endurance, it would be just over a second in both directions of the movement at a 1.25-to-1.25 second count.

Muscular Size (Hypertrophy)

I'm confident that if you're reading this book, you're primarily interested in honoring God with your body rather than creating "body beautiful." However, you may have sustained an injury to an area of your body, requiring rebuilding. Here is a good way to exercise to increase muscle size.

Repetitions per Exercise

To increase the size of muscle, use a moderate level of resistance, at a moderate number of repetitions, at a uniform and slow speed of movement. Your objective in increasing muscle size is to affect the center areas of the muscle, not the tapered ends. Focus on the repetitions, not the weight being lifted, nor jerking in your movements.

Repeat movements at least eight times, but not more than fifteen. Most trainers will have you perform ten to twelve repetitions in a controlled movement to the point of complete exhaustion in every set.

Sets per Exercise

The total number of sets to increase muscular size is similar to strength development. Perform at least four sets, but not more than seven. Most trainers will have you perform five sets to get as much blood and oxygen into that muscle as possible. The whole idea is to break down the structural integrity of the muscle without actually injuring it so that it is forced to adapt to the imposed stress by getting larger. The extent to which your muscles can enlarge is determined by your genes. But everyone can enlarge his or her muscles to that point.

Speed of Movement

The key to enlarging muscle is slowing down the movement so that the intramuscular tension can rise to the highest level. To do this, the weight lifted will be lighter than in strength development.

You may have heard that you should make your movements "super slow." This isn't true. Moving super slowly requires too light of a resistance. To increase muscle size, go for a two-to-two count. Two seconds raising the weight, and two seconds in lowering the weight. Trust me, this will seem very slow. Enjoy!

The Pre-exhaust Training Concept

I want to introduce you to pre-exhaust training for your strength development. This concept makes total sense. Always perform the largest muscle group and body movements first, and the smaller muscles and movements last. This is because when you're exercising your upper back, for example, you're also using your arms by way of your biceps. And, when you're working your chest muscles, you'll also be using your triceps (the back of your upper arm). If you exercise your arms and legs before your back, chest, hips, and core, respectively, you'll already be too fatigued to do a good job in conditioning the biggest muscles and joints in your body. So, here's the order I recommend you perform your exercises:

Upper Body

1. Upper Back
2. Chest
3. Shoulders
4. Arms

Lower Body

1. Hips (glutes, lower back, hip flexors, and upper thigh)
2. Core (mid, side, and upper abdominals, mid-to-lower back)
3. Legs (mid-to-lower thigh, calf, ankle)

The Ascending Pyramid

I may be overwhelming you with these exercise facts, but remember: knowledge will empower you. You'll be more likely to persevere if you understand the whys and the hows. This next concept is critical to your success and safety.

The Lord installed protective mechanisms in your brain to prevent injury. He did this in part by installing a protection mechanism called *physical and mental inhibition.* This simply means the brain and the body will hold back effort, intensity, and movements until they're sure that it's safe before giving themselves totally to something. This is the main reason you have to perform multiple sets. This is also why you can't just go to the heaviest weight and try to lift it. Your brain won't let you. And, if you try anyway, you'll probably hurt yourself. This happened to me back in 1976. I didn't warm into the lifting sequence properly before I attempted to perform a 400-pound barbell dead lift. I injured my lower back badly for a while. We have to use the common sense the Lord gave us, the "sound mind" Paul spoke of in 2 Timothy 1:7. When I'm strength training someone to develop their back, chest, hips and upper thighs, I have them perform their exercises in a five-set protocol.

"Knowledge will empower you."

- First set is lightweight for twelve repetitions.
- Second set we add some weight and perform ten repetitions.
- Third set we add more weight and perform eight repetitions. At this point, there is already a fair amount of strain involved.
- Fourth set we add additional weight and strain to get barely six repetitions.
- If you feel safe, we add the most weight possible for a fifth set, limiting your repetitions to three or four, or until complete muscular failure.

This is the safe way to increase your strength over time, especially if you're a beginner. When you're first starting out, perform the first three sets at twelve, ten, and eight repetitions, respectively. Also perform these three sets and repetitions for smaller muscle groups, such as the shoulders, upper arms, and calves. There is greater risk of injury to these vulnerable joints and muscle groups if you lift too heavy a weight.

Before I give you a great strength workout that you can perform anywhere in the world using minimal equipment, I want you to know the hierarchy—a rating of strength exercises from the best to the lesser ones. I want you functionally strong so you can carry out the Lord's purpose in your life.

Internal Resistance

Internal resistance uses your own body weight to develop strength as well as joint flexibility and body elasticity. This type of exercise will always be superior because, after all, it is your *body.* Body weight exercise goes very deep, strengthening your tendons, ligaments, and other connective tissues. You can create an almost unlimited variety of body resistance movements. Military forces are masters at internal resistance exercises, especially elite units such as the U.S. Navy SEAL teams.

To top it off, internal resistance body weight exercise produces a body that is strong, light, and close to the bone. I perform internal resistance exercise before literally all workouts. I know to make these movements my priority.

External Resistance

External resistance involves exerting force against resistance from outside your body. The Lord created our bodies to pick things up, to move, throw, or kick them. He also created the physical law of gravity. That which goes straight up, unless another force is exerted against it, will come straight down. So, a ten-pound weight will always weigh ten pounds, no matter what plane of motion it is in, or how much leverage you have over it.

Lifting weight that is free, unattached, and movable, goes according to nature. And this is why free-weight barbells, dumbbells, or anything that can provide resistance, such as a rock, board, or paint can, is the next best way to improve your strength and performance.

External Resistance Exercise Machines

Performing strength exercise on resistance machines that load weight plates, weight stacks, and use cables and pulleys are still beneficial for you, but they are limited in simulating the myriad of movements you use in real life. Exercise machines perform specific movements and joint actions. They provide resistance against primary muscles, but they don't develop all of the helper muscles. A plus for these machines is that the learning curve is low. Also, they help you not hurt yourself. Most professional trainers, including myself, use exercise machines here and there in our workouts, if they're available.

External Resistance Rubber Tubing

External resistance training with latex rubber tubing has become very popular. It is very useful in physical therapy and can be advantageous for traveling, as you can pack them in your suitcase. However, the Lord didn't create our bodies to deal with resistance that changes as it lengthens or shortens. The Lord created the law of gravity with free weight objects that weigh the same, no matter how much leverage you have over them. Still, most of us do use rubber tubing now and then in our workouts, just not exclusively.

	Benefit Hierarchy
Superior	Internal resistance exercise using body weight • Pull-ups • Chins • Pushups • Dips • Hanging body curls
Excellent	External resistance using free weight equipment • Barbells • Dumbbells • Paint cans • Wooden planks
Good	External resistance using machine apparatus • Specific body part machines • Pulleys and cables • Various style benches
Fair	External resistance using latex rubber tubing and bungee cords

Figure 12.2 Hierarchy of functional strength exercise

Additional Concepts

Recovery between Sets

When I first start strength-training work with a beginner, he or she tends to feel the need to rush through a workout. But remember: when we're strength training, we're not concerned about aerobic conditioning. So there's no need to be in a hurry. In fact, if you don't take the adequate rest between your sets, you're actually taking away from the benefits of the workout. There are two primary reasons to take an official rest between your sets of resistance exercise.

1. The nerves and muscles need time to refuel with ATP.
2. The nerves and muscles need time to assimilate potassium, sodium, calcium, and magnesium (these are the contractile minerals).

The amount of rest is dependent upon a number of factors—your mood, how much sleep you've been getting, how you've been eating, and the intensity of your present exercise. Here's a rule of thumb: when you feel like your breathing and heart rate have returned to a relatively restful state and your muscles feel like they've recovered, it's time for another set. Generally, you should rest from ninety seconds to two minutes between your sets. But above all, listen to your body.

Exercise Breathing

I often get a real kick out of it when my clients ask me, "How should I be breathing as I perform this set of exercise?"

I reply, "You should breathe in and breathe out." Seriously though, people ask this because they've read or heard about breathing a certain way from somewhere. Medical experts came up with special breathing technique for people with serious coronary heart and vascular disease. For the healthy person, holding your breath is a natural response to the strain of any movement. When I run sprints, I hold my breath on and off over the distance run. Holding your breath causes something like a pneumatic air back brace, stabilizing your lower back and core, facilitating unrestricted movement and speed of your arms and legs. It's productive as long as you're relatively healthy.

When you hold your breath as you're straining, you invoke the Valsalva maneuver. The Valsalva maneuver is a response to strain. This breath holding causes the blood to stay in your skull and not return down to the heart for reoxygenation and recirculation. If an individual has coronary heart risk factors such as smoking, high blood pressure, high cholesterol, high triglycerides, and excessive body fat, this high buildup of pressure could dislodge a blood clot or stop the heart altogether. So in these cases, it is a good idea not to hold your breath and overstrain. Proper breathing would be to inhale through your nose and mouth while lowering the weight, extending a limb, or relaxing between repetitions. You would then breathe out through your mouth between pursed lips while lifting the weight or straining to overcome the resistance in that particular moment.

So, are you ready for your anyplace strength workout? Say yes and amen!

The Anyplace Strength Workout

I've designed this anyplace strength workout for the person on the go, and for the one who doesn't have a fitness facility available. It's nothing fancy, but it'll get the job done. Please consider drinking eight ounces of pure water before your workout begins, and then drink an additional eight ounces of water every fifteen minutes during the workout. Let's start out by doing a few calisthenics to warm up and prepare the joints of your body.

Jumping Jacks

First, assume the standard starting position: feet hip-width apart, knees slightly bent, hands on your hips, shoulders back and down, and abdominals in. Then in one motion, jump upward while simultaneously extending your feet outward approximately six inches, and bringing your hands together over your head. Jump back with feet together and hands at your sides. Perform one set of thirty repetitions.

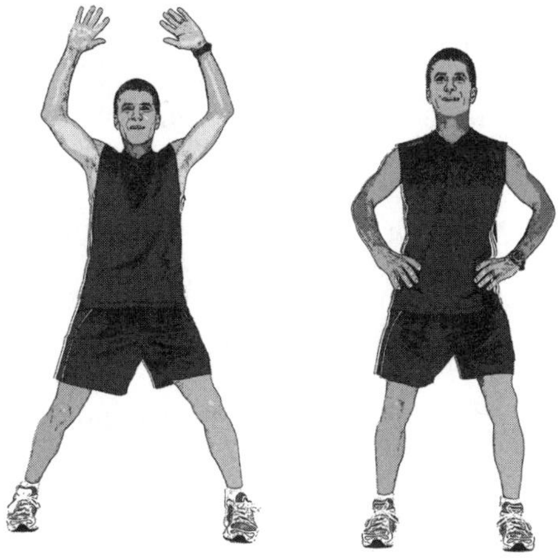

FIGURE 12.3 JUMPING JACKS

Rotary Twists

This is a great movement to loosen up your shoulders and lower back. Assume standard starting position. Keep your arms up in front of you at chest height. Begin gently rotating to your left and then to your right. Make sure to keep a slight bend in your knees. Perform forty repetitions of twenty to the left and twenty to the right for one set.

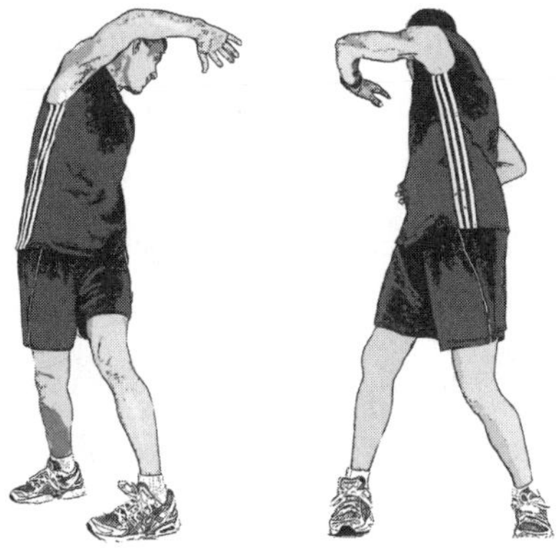

FIGURE 12.4 ROTARY TWISTS

Body Weight Squats

This one will stretch your lower back while warming up your hips and knees. Assume a standard starting position. Turn your toes slightly outward so that, when you squat down, your knees follow your toes. As you keep your head up and your back neutral, squat down and simultaneously extend your arms down in front of you with your palms up. Perform one set of thirty repetitions.

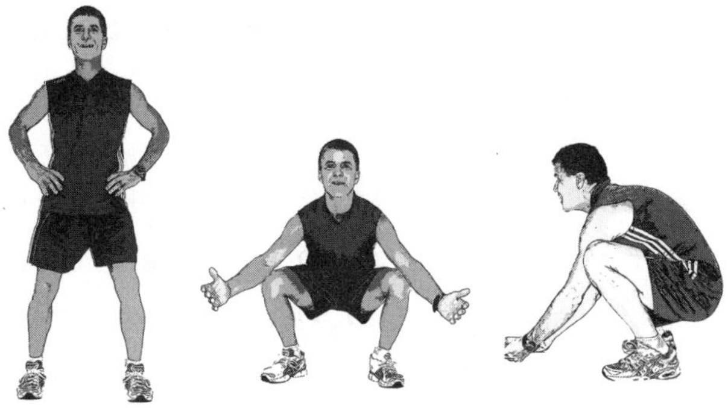

FIGURE 12.5 BODY WEIGHT SQUATS

Side Bends

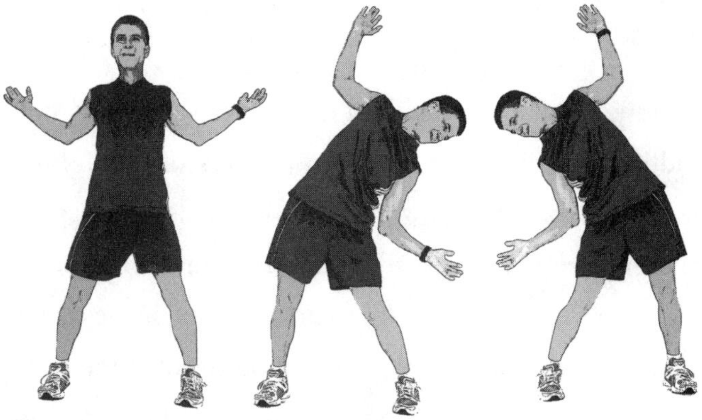

Figure 12.6 Side bends

Here's another one to warm up your side, lower back, and hips. Assume a standard starting position, but with your arms extended up and your shoulders back. Bend to your left until your left elbow touches your left hip. Come back upright and then over to your right side. Perform one set of forty repetitions, twenty to your left and twenty to your right.

Alternating Toe Touches

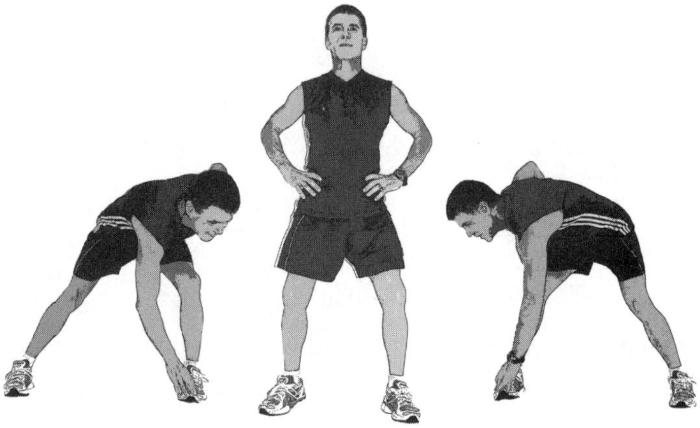

Figure 12.7 Alternating toe touches

This classic, whole body movement is going to finish the warm-up and get you into your workout. Assume the standard starting position. Throughout this movement, make sure to keep flexing at the knees. Bend over and touch your right hand to your left foot. Now straighten up, then bend over to your right side in a fluid, sweeping motion. Perform one set of thirty repetitions, alternating for a total of fifteen to the left and fifteen to the right.

Bent-Over Row

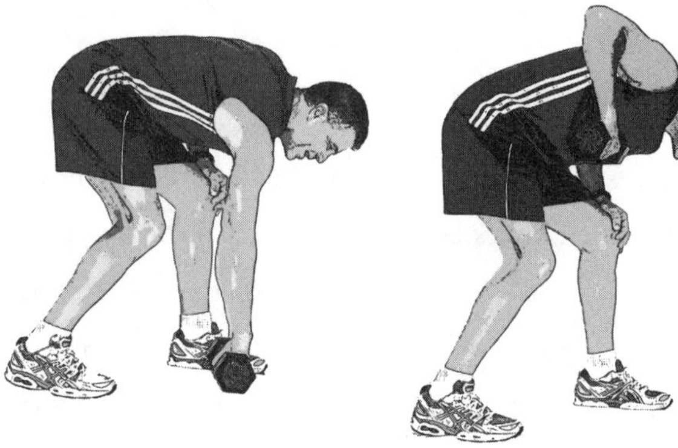

Figure 12.8 Bent-over row

Find something you can place your left hand on, such as a chair or bench. Pick up a dumbbell, paint can, or other object that weighs five to twenty pounds. Place it on the ground in front of the bench. Bend over and place your left hand on the bench. Grab the weight in your right hand while assuming a stance with your right foot forward and your left foot back. Keep your back flat and parallel with the ground. Pull the weight straight up to your chest as you extend your elbow to your outside. Lower the weight down to the ground at a one-second count. Perform your first set of twelve repetitions for your right side and then your left side. For your second set, try to slightly increase the weight you're lifting and perform ten repetitions for your right and left sides. If possible, try to increase the weight again for your third set. Perform eight repetitions for your right and left sides. Remember that, by your last set, you should experience a fair amount of muscular strain. This exercise works your upper back and back of your shoulders.

Pushups

Using a bench or something that elevates your hand position decreases the resistance of this movement. The lower you are to the ground, the higher the resistance. Assume a shoulder-width hand position where your arms are extended and your spine is neutral. While keeping your elbows out, lower your chest to the edge of the bench or to the ground. Push your body back up to an arms-extended position. Perform as many quality repetitions as possible at a one-to-one count. Do three sets. This exercise works your chest, front shoulders, and the back of your upper arms.

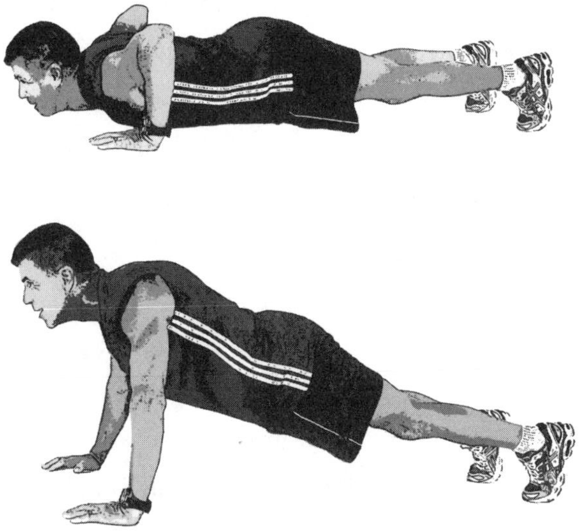

FIGURE 12.9 PUSHUP

Upright Row

Find something that you can hang onto with both hands, and that weighs at least twenty pounds. Pick up the weight with an overhand grip. Assume the standard starting position. Pull your hands straight up to shoulder height as you extend your elbows straight up. Perform twelve repetitions on your first set. As always, if you can go up in weight from set to set, do so. Otherwise, just make sure you get a good strain at least on your third and last set. Repetition sets are twelve, ten, and eight. This is probably the best exercise for your neck and upper shoulder muscles.

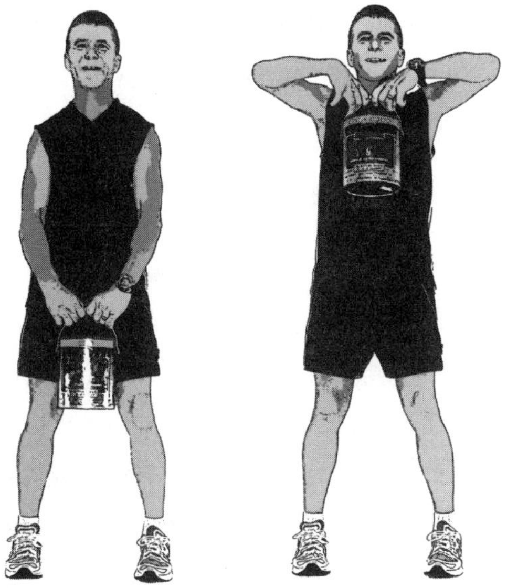

FIGURE 12.10 UPRIGHT ROW

Shoulder Press

This is another great shoulder exercise, but instead of pulling, you're pushing straight overhead. Find two equal weights of at least ten pounds, or locate a board or something you can grip at a shoulder-width hand position. Assume the standard starting position. Pull the weight up to the start position, even with the top of your chest. While keeping your head forward, press the weight straight overhead with your arms extended. Perform sets of twelve, ten, and eight repetitions.

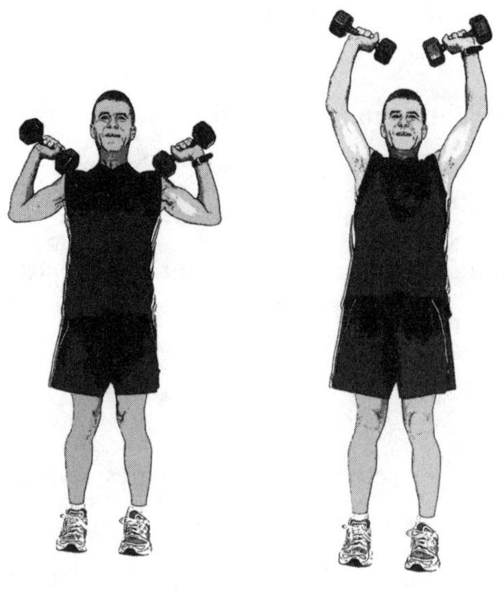

Figure 12.11 Shoulder press

Biceps Curls

This exercise works your front upper arm and the inside of your forearm. Find equal weights of at least ten pounds for each arm, or a board or branch that weighs twenty pounds. Now assume standard starting position. With your hands in an underhand position, flex your elbow and lift your hands to your front shoulders. Extend your arms back down to your side. Perform sets of twelve, ten, and eight repetitions.

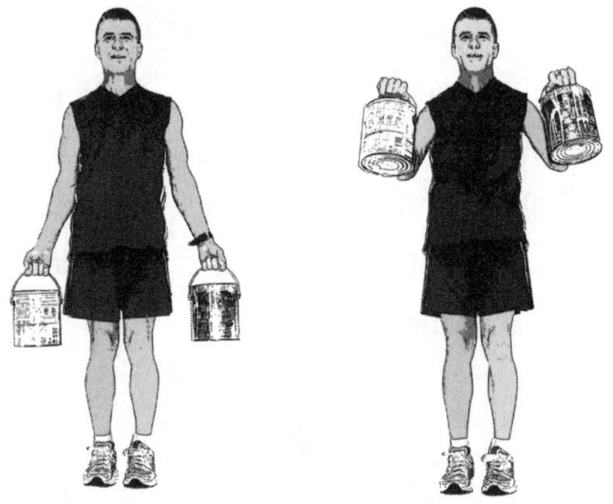

Figure 12.12 Biceps curls

Squats

Okay. We're ready to work your core and lower body. We're going back to the squat, like you did in the warm-up, except now you're going to add resistance of at least twenty pounds in each hand. As you perform your squats, keep your head up and your spine neutral. Hold your arms at your side. Perform sets of twelve, ten, and eight repetitions. This exercise is the best for your hips, thighs, and core.

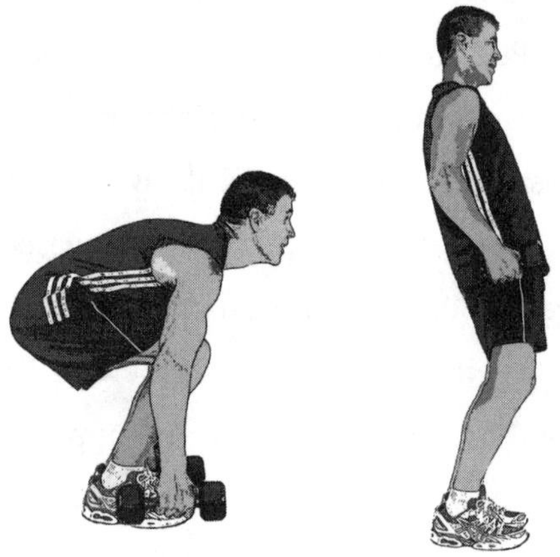

Figure 12.13 Squats

Crunches

Let's get those abdominals while saving your lower back. Lie down on the ground with your spine in a neutral position against the surface. Bend your knees forty-five degrees with your feet flat on the ground. Put your fingertips lightly behind your head. As you look straight up, contract your abdominal muscles and lift your head, neck, and shoulders as one unit. Make sure to keep your back on the ground. Perform sets of fifteen, twenty, and twenty-five repetitions.

Lateral Lunge

This exercise will tone the inside of your legs, especially the upper thigh. Find something that weighs at least twenty pounds. Assume a wider-than-standard starting position. Keeping your head up and lower back in a neutral position, straighten your left leg and go into a single right leg squat position. Return to upright and move to your left side. Perform sets of twelve, ten, and eight repetitions, going right and left for each leg and hip.

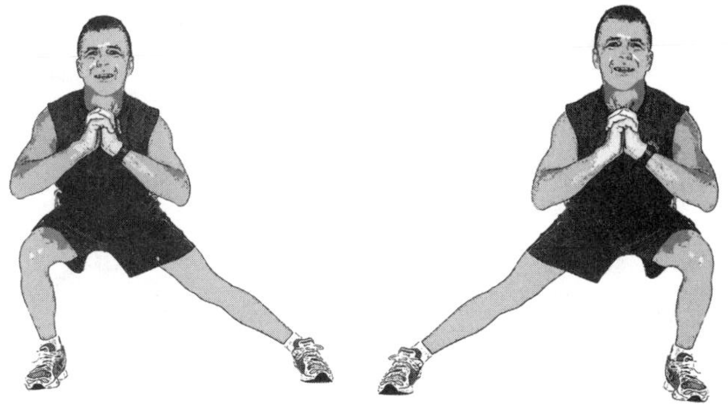

Figure 12.14 Lateral lunge

Side Bend

Let's get rid of those love handles and trim your waist. Find a fifteen-pound weight. Assume a foot position where your legs are stiff and your feet are together. With the weight in your right hand, dip sideways to your right, and then side bend as far as you can to your left. Perform one set to your left for twenty repetitions, and then twenty to your right with the weight in your left hand. Increase your weight by five pounds, and then perform a set of fifteen repetitions to your left and then your right.

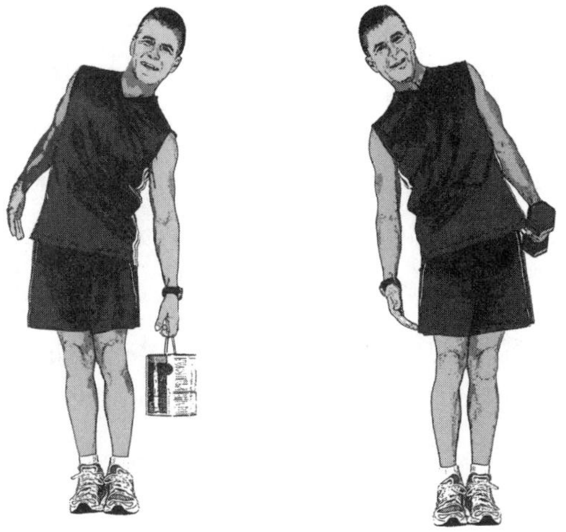

Figure 12.15 Side bend

Stiff-Leg Dead Lift

We finish the workout with an exercise that works your buttocks and the backs of your thighs. It also stretches and pulls in your abdominal muscles. Find a board or something that weighs at least twenty pounds. Assume the starting position but keep your knees locked straight. While keeping your head up and your back flat, bend down to the ground until you feel your knees wanting to bend. Straighten up to the standing position. Perform sets of twelve, ten, and eight repetitions.

After your strength building workout, I recommend you perform some static stretches to help prevent soreness and improve your flexibility. An excellent static stretch routine is provided in the next chapter.

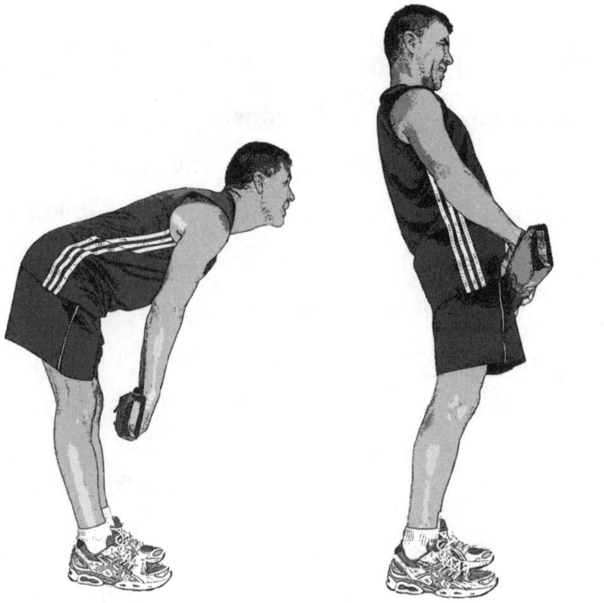

FIGURE 12.16 STIFF-LEG DEAD LIFT

Anaerobic Sprint Workouts

You'll remember that I said not to condition your heart, lungs, and circulatory pathways at an intensity greater than 75 percent of your predicted maximum heart rate. I also said that I was going to max out your heart rate for an anaerobic benefit later. Now is that time. Running sprints is a one-stop shop to exercise all of your 206 bones and 650 muscles at the same time. Initially, the intensity of a sprint will seem bizarre. You'll feel like your lungs are going to explode and your heart is going to burst out of your chest. But as you emotionally and physically adapt to this unparalleled intensity, you'll realize that this exercise has the biggest bang for your buck. You'll find yourself making sprints a priority. Thirty to forty minutes of sprints at least two to three days per week will accelerate your body fat/body mass reduction while anabolically increasing your strength, power, and muscularity. I've said it before, that to me sprints are an act of worship. I'm closest to the Lord when I'm at my physical maximum. I think the Lord loves physicality. Jesus was a carpenter and worked vigorously at his trade. There's no doubt in my mind that in some way Jesus' hard work growing up helped him endure the cross.

Getting Started

Your sprint mechanics are as follows:

1. Run with your feet hip-width apart, like they are on separate train tracks, and your toes straight ahead.

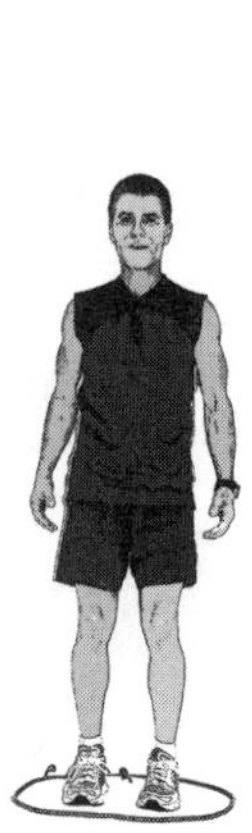

FIGURE 12.17 FEET HIP-WIDTH APART

2. As you sprint, keep a good bend in your knees. Have your foot strike on the center of the ball of your foot only (no heel strike).
3. Make sure that your foot strike lands straight below your hips. Keep your arms and shoulders at a ninety-degree joint angle. As you sprint, flex and extend your arms from the point of your shoulder. At the downstroke, your relaxed hands are even with your back pocket. On the upstroke, your hands are even with your jaw and lined up with your ear on the respective side of your body.

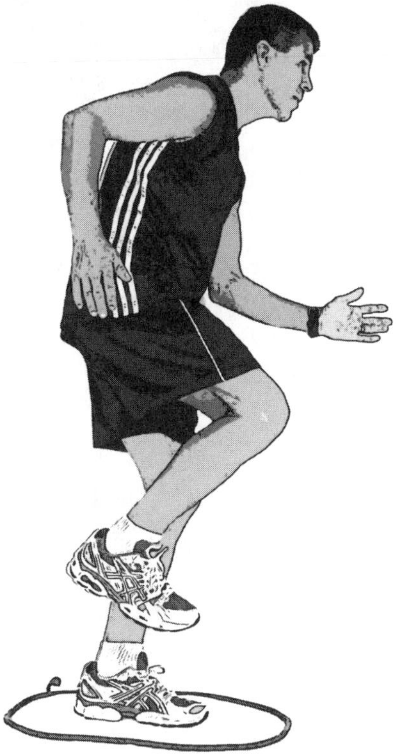

FIGURE 12.18 FEET UNDER HIPS AND NINETY-DEGREE ARM ANGLE

4. As you sprint, pull your heel straight up under your body by using your hamstring and buttocks muscles. Fall gently forward and let your feet fall lightly under your hip. Treat the ground surface as white-hot coals.

Here's a realistic sprint workout sequence. Start by running ten sixty-yard buildup sprints. A buildup sprint begins as a jog, rises to a sprint, then decreases back to a jog at completion. Rest as much as you need to recover your breath between sprints. Perform these sprints at least two days a week and not more than four days apart. Over the weeks to come, increase your sprint distances to one hundred yards and your number of sprints to twenty. Once you can consistently run twenty hundred-yard sprints at least three days per week, increase your overall effort and intensity, but add no additional sprints. Your exercise intensity should be at 90 to 100 percent.

Consider twenty-five meter swim sprints as a variance to your running sprints if you have body issues that prevent you from running the ground-based sprints.

Recreational Ground-Based Sports

I recommend that whenever possible you play competitive, ground-based sports to maintain your coordination, balance, agility, and quickness. The random chaos associated with being forced to respond fast mentally is also great exercise for your brain. Sports such as tennis, soccer, and basketball are lifetime sports that people of both genders and all ages can play. Here's a list of sports you might have fun playing:

- Soccer
- Basketball
- Volleyball
- Touch football
- Frisbee

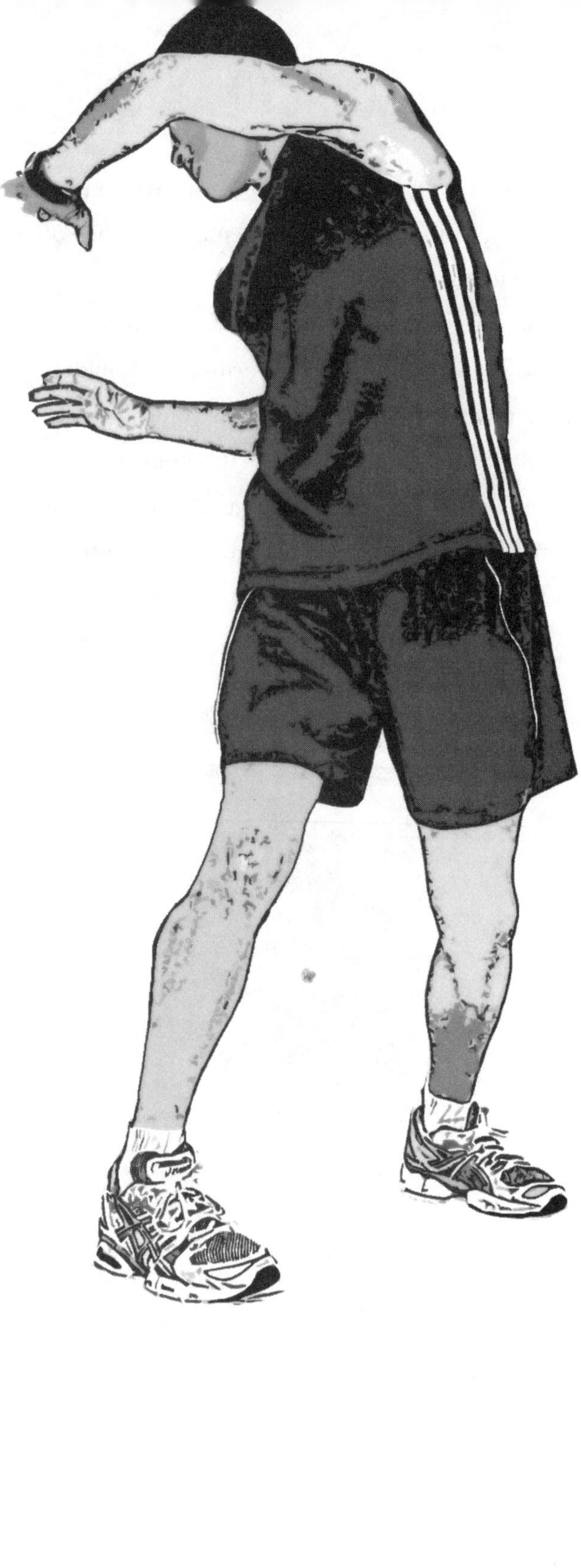

Overtraining Symptoms

Be aware of becoming emotionally and physically addicted to your exercise. Don't make it an idol—the Lord won't have it. He has put physical laws in place that will tell you when you're overdoing it and when it's time to back off. Here are some indicators:

- If you used to look forward to your workouts but now find yourself dreading the next one.
- You feel overly fatigued with a heaviness of limbs.
- You're more irritable.
- You're weak when you should be strong in your movements.
- Your muscles and joints are aching more than normal after workouts.
- You feel flu-like symptoms.
- You've sustained some sort of inflammatory tendonitis in one or more of your joints.
- You're having trouble getting a good night's sleep.

Let's now move to an important part of physical fitness, which is often neglected—joint flexibility and body elasticity.

>> *tip:* Eat and Move

Have a small glass of organic vegetable juice. I like it hot and spicy because it gives me some pizzazz. You'll raise your metabolic rate and satisfy a couple of your fruit and vegetable serving with this snack.

13

JOINT FLEXIBILITY AND BODY ELASTICITY

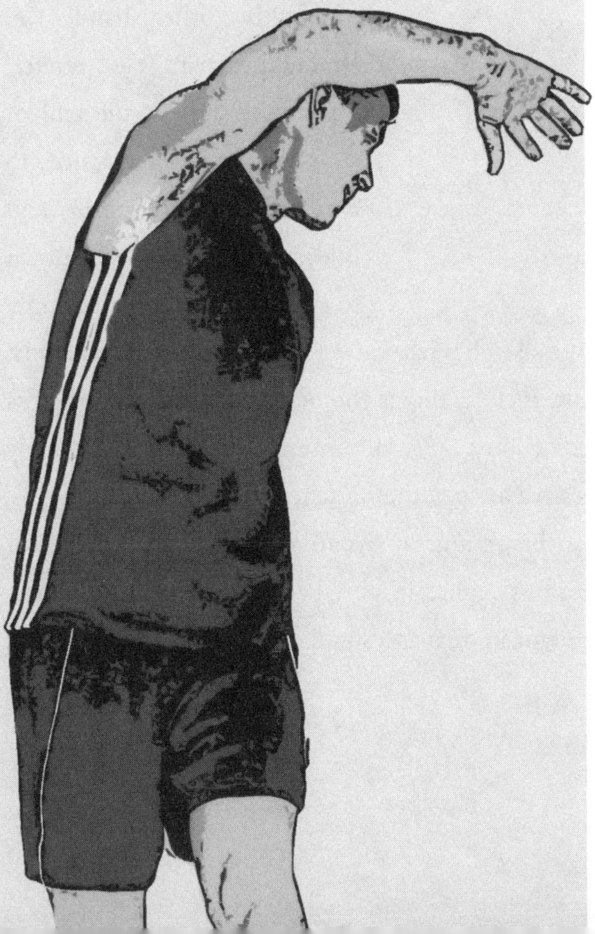

Flexibility and body elasticity development is the most neglected component in physical fitness, especially at the end of one's workout. Most of us have hectic schedules, so just fitting our aerobic or strength workout in is hard enough. But we must include this component of fitness into our weekly workouts. As a physical fitness professional who trains three hours a day, six days per week, even I know that I should be making flexibility and elasticity training more of a priority.

Flexibility and Elasticity Defined

Body flexibility is your body's ability to move unrestrictedly through your joints' ranges of motion. It's the absence of tightness in your movements. Related terms include mobility, pliability, and suppleness.

Elasticity simply means that, after something is stretched, it has the ability to return to its original shape. A rubber band is a classic example of elasticity. The energy that propels a rubber band through the air is simply its returning to its original shape before it was stretched and released. Related terms include springiness and twistability.

Dr. Laurence E. Morehouse, the man who designed the astronaut fitness training program, also wrote an incredible book that changed my life. It's titled *Maximum Performance.** He presents fifteen movement principles to improve physical performance in any endeavor. One principle is that in any human movement we should have our body relaxed but together, taut but not tight. We need to have just the right amount of tension within our body at any given time. He refers to it as "optimal anxiety."

* Laurence E. Morehouse, PhD, and Leonard Gross, *Maximum Performance* (New York: Simon & Schuster, 1977).

The primary method we use to improve flexibility and elasticity is various stretching movements. An added benefit is that stretching also increases body strength and muscle tone. As you elongate a joint and stretch the muscles, tension is loaded into the system. Thus, muscle tone is increased and your ability to exert more force is improved. Remember, everything in your body was designed by the Lord to work together for the good of the whole.

Types of Flexibility and Elasticity

When most people think of flexibility, they might picture track and field athletes who are sprawled out on the grass performing stretches for their groin and hamstring muscles. Static or stationary stretches like these are one form of stretching to improve flexibility. Another is dynamic stretching, where you're performing some of the same movements as in your workout but at a much lower intensity. It's an *easing into* your movements to prevent injury and maximize the quality and benefits of your training.

"Remember, everything in your body was designed by the Lord to work together for the good of the whole."

Both stationary and dynamic stretching are excellent. The type you choose depends on your circumstances. What are you about to do in your workout? Where are you in that workout? Are you at the beginning, middle, or end of that activity? These answers determine which flexibility exercises you should choose.

Specificity of Exercise

One common sense concept is "specificity of exercise." Specificity of exercise says simply, if you want to develop some form of physical fitness, you have to train specifically in *that form.* Seems obvious, doesn't it? How do you improve in basketball? By playing basketball, of course. You wouldn't try to improve in basketball by playing tennis, would you? Yet countless coaches, trainers, and exercisers fail to understand this. They're constantly having people do movements that aren't remotely related to improving in a specific activity.

So, if you're training for a dynamic movement, then your warm-up should also be dynamic. By performing movements directly related to the workout activity, you're actually giving your brain time to adapt and get the entire body involved. Dynamic flexibility exercises prepare the brain and the body for the actual exercise or sport.

On the other hand, you should perform static stretching movements at the end of your workouts or practices to decompress your brain and body, to bring them back down to a relaxed state. The best time for static stretch is when the body is warmed up and most resilient. In fact, this is the best time to make progress in specific joint range of motion, especially if you apply progressive force in the stretches.

Now, here's a great dynamic flexibility workout you can perform either in part before a strength or sports workout, or in total as a stand-alone workout.

The Calisthenic Strength and Body Elasticity Workout

You can do this workout anywhere. You don't need special equipment, other than maybe a bench seat for two of the exercises. This is an internal resistance, body-weight workout of eighteen different exercises. Going through all eighteen exercises will take twenty to twenty-five minutes. Generally, I go through all eighteen exercises twice for a forty-five minute workout. I have lots of friends who absolutely love this workout. I hope you will, too.

Jumping Jacks

Assume the standard starting position with your hands on your hips. Jump straight up as you spread your feet apart six inches to the outside. Simultaneously bring your hands together over your head. Jump back with feet together and hands at your side. This is a great whole body exercise. Perform thirty repetitions on your first set and forty repetitions on your second.

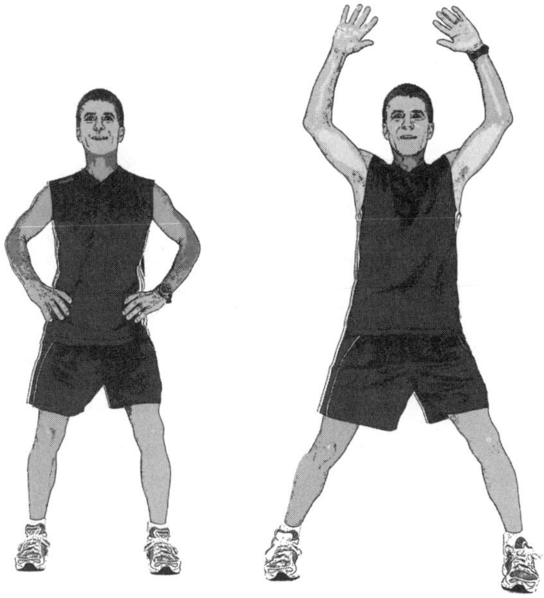

FIGURE 13.1 JUMPING JACKS

Body Weight Squats

Assume starting position with your hands on your hips. Keep your head up and your lower back slightly arched as you squat down. Turn your toes slightly to the outside and have your knees follow your toes as you squat down. Return to the starting position. This is a great exercise for your hips, core, and thighs. Perform twenty repetitions on your first set, and twenty-five on your second.

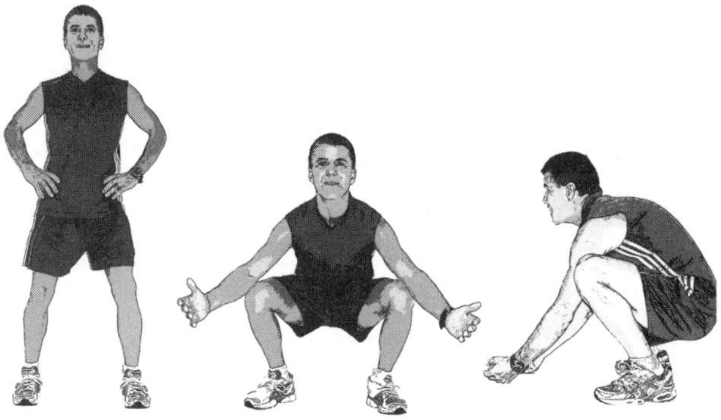

FIGURE 13.2 BODY WEIGHT SQUATS

Rotary Twists

This is great for your abdominals and lower back. Assume a hip-width foot position with your arms in front of you at chest height. Gently rotate to your left and to your right. Make sure to keep a slight bend in your knees to keep your lower back relaxed. Perform thirty repetitions left and right for your first set, and forty for your second set.

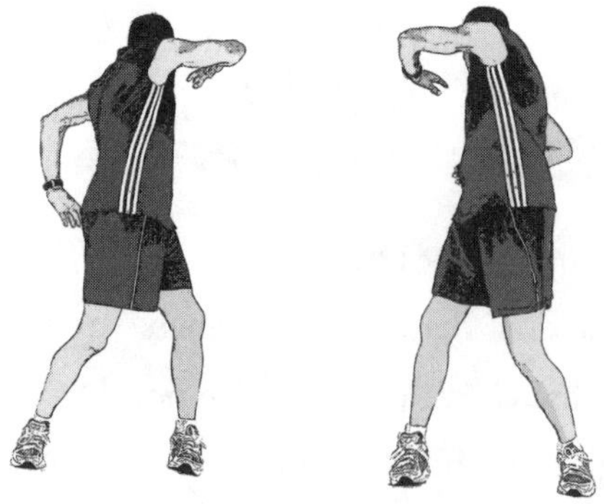

FIGURE 13.3 ROTARY TWISTS

Twist and Jump

This is a fun whole body exercise. Start by assuming a hip-width foot position and turn your lower body forty-five degrees to the left. Turn your upper body forty-five degrees to the right. Jump up and rotate your foot position to the right and your arms to the left. Perform thirty repetitions left and right on the first set, and forty on the second.

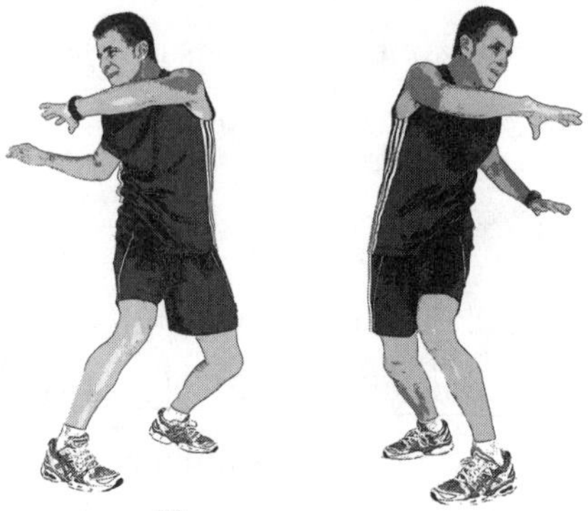

FIGURE 13.4 TWIST AND JUMP

Side Bends

This will work the sides of your lower back and love handles. Assume the starting position. Staying upright, bend to your left, touching your left elbow to your left hip, and then over to your right. Remember to always keep a bend in your knees. Perform thirty repetitions left and right on the first set, and forty on the second.

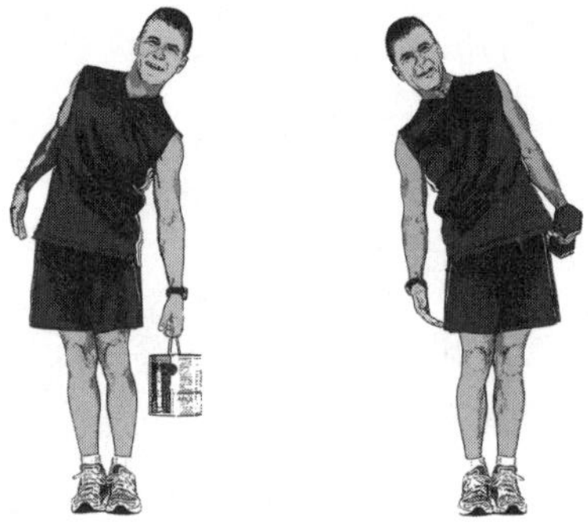

FIGURE 13.5 SIDE BENDS

Skaters

Here is one for your inner thighs and outside hips. Assume a foot position much wider than hip-width. Begin by jumping to your left while swinging your right arm up until your hand is even with your jaw. Then jump right. Perform thirty repetitions left and right on the first set, and forty on the second.

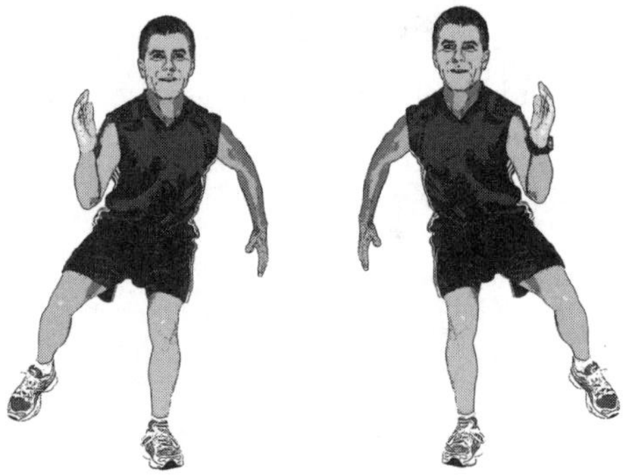

FIGURE 13.6 SKATERS

High Knee Raises

This lower abdominal exercise will also stretch your lower back. Assume the starting position. Balance on your right foot as you lift your left knee up as high as possible. Simultaneously swing your right arm and hand up even with your jaw. Then lift your right knee, swinging your left arm up. Perform thirty repetitions left and right on the first set, then forty on the second.

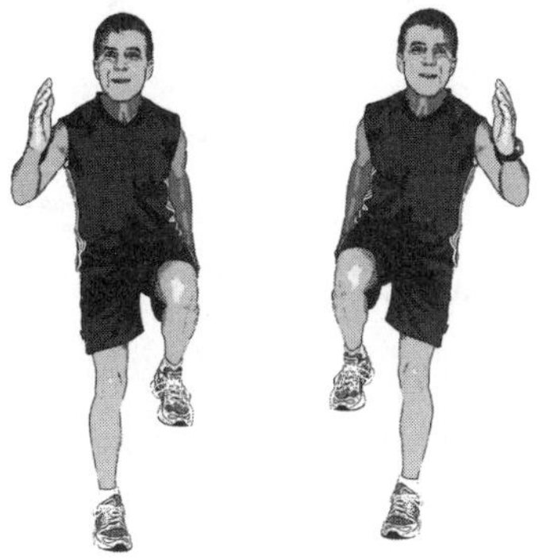

FIGURE 13.7 HIGH KNEE RAISES

Alternating Toe Touches

This is my favorite calisthenic exercise. It's a classic that works your hips, core, and legs. Assume a foot position slightly wider than hip-width with your hands on your hips and knees slightly bent. Bend down and touch your right hand to your left foot, then switch sides, touching your left hand to your right foot. Perform thirty repetitions left and right on your first set, and forty on your second set.

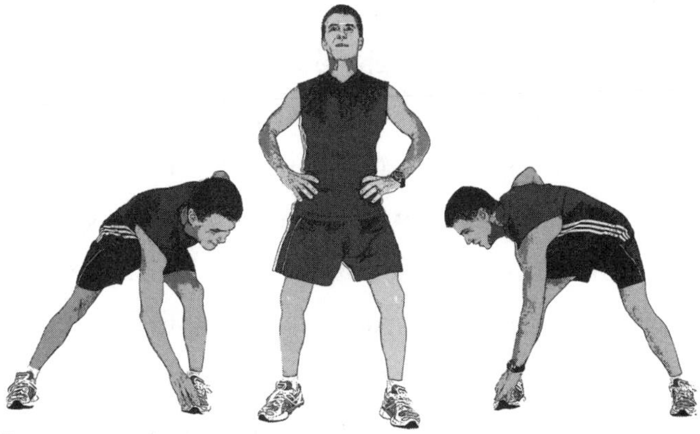

FIGURE 13.8 ALTERNATING TOE TOUCHES

Lateral Lunge Squats

Here is one to tone the inside of your leg from the ankle to the groin. Assume a very wide foot position with your hands folded together in front of your chest. While keeping your upper body straight and upright, straighten your right leg as you slide laterally to your left into a single-leg squat position. Then slide right. Perform thirty repetitions left and right on the first set, and forty on the second.

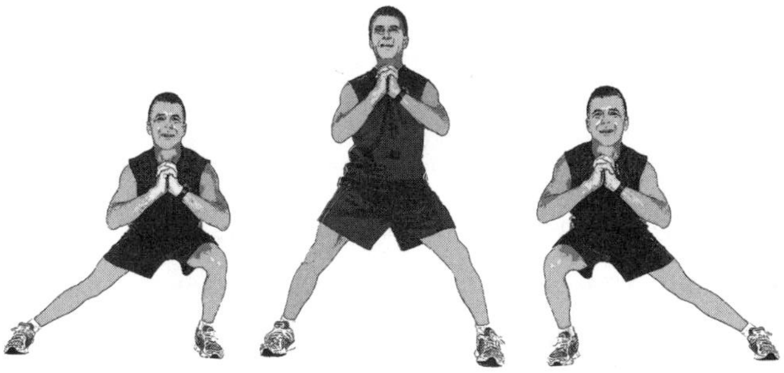

FIGURE 13.9 LATERAL LUNGE SQUATS

Lying Leg Raises

While also strengthening your lower back, this exercise really works that lower abdomen. Sit on the floor, extend your legs in front, and lean back on your elbows with your palms flat on the floor. Put a slight bend in your knee and lift your legs straight up about a foot, then slowly lower them back down. Perform twenty repetitions on the first set, and twenty-five on the second set.

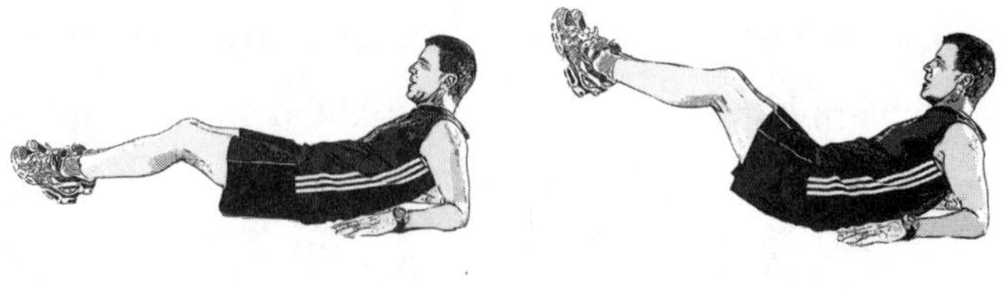

FIGURE 13.10 LYING LEG RAISES

Pushups

These will work your chest, shoulders, and arms. Lie face down on the floor. Position your hands shoulder width apart, with your palms flat against the floor. Hold your core stable and get up on your toes. Press straight up to the arms-extended position. While looking straight ahead, slowly lower and touch your chest to the ground. Use a bench seat if you need to decrease the resistance. Perform as many quality repetitions on the first set as possible, and then perform the same number or more on the second set.

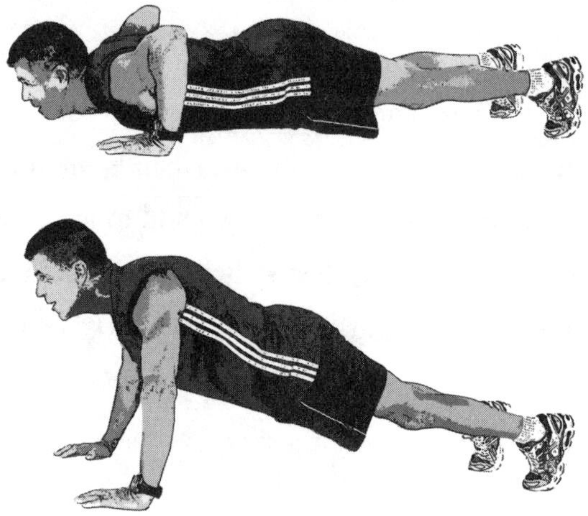

FIGURE 13.11 PUSHUPS

Pull-down Squeeze

Strengthen the upper back and shoulders while stretching the chest with this movement. Assume a hip-width foot stance and extend your arms over your head. Pull your elbows straight down and back, squeezing your back muscles. Reach back up, and perform twenty repetitions on your first set and twenty-five on your second.

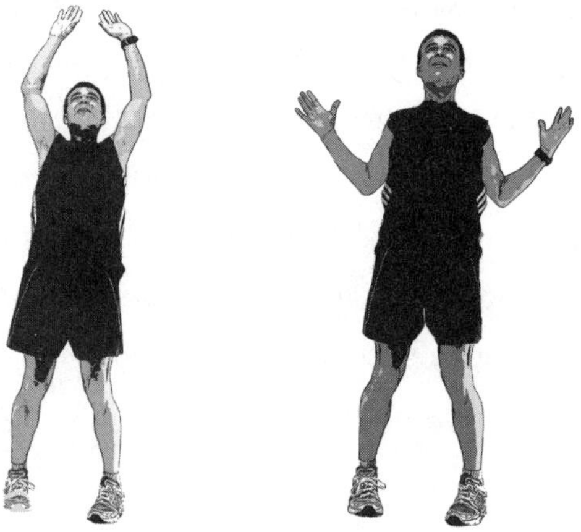

FIGURE 13.12 PULL-DOWN SQUEEZE

Touchdown Lunges

This exercise works the top of your shoulders, your ribs, core, and the back of your thighs. Assume the starting position with your hands on your hips. Step forward with your left foot as deep as possible, and lower your right knee gently to the ground. Simultaneously extend your arms straight up over your head and signal "touchdown" or "goal." From there, drive your body weight back up into the start position, and step right. Perform twenty repetitions left and right on the first set, and thirty on the second set.

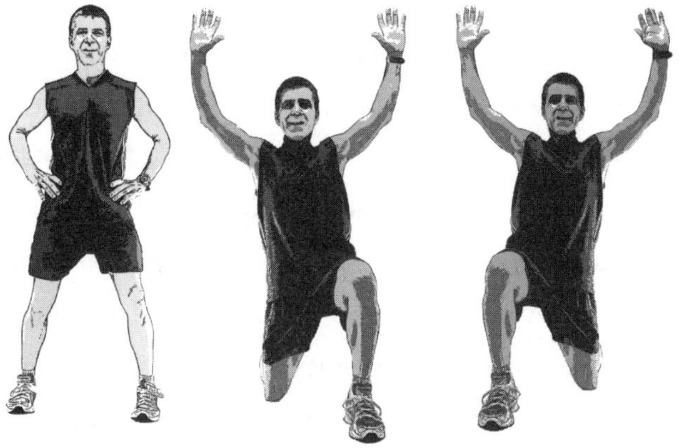

FIGURE 13.13 TOUCHDOWN LUNGES

Thumbs-up Rows

This will improve the posture of your upper middle back and rear shoulders. Assume a hip-width starting position. Extend your arms straight in front and round your back forward like a cat. Pull your elbows straight back and together as you turn your thumbs straight up. Perform twenty repetitions on your first set, and twenty-five on the second.

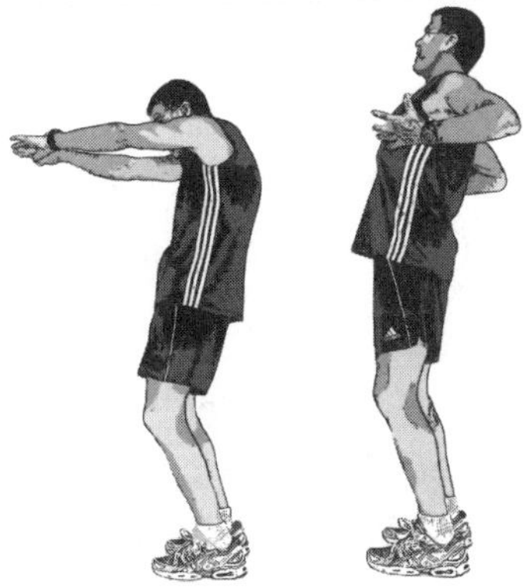

FIGURE 13.14 THUMBS-UP ROWS

Split Jumps

Although this is a whole body exercise, it really hits the thighs and the calves. Assume the starting position. Now step forward with your left foot while you raise your right arm up with your hand even with your jaw. This is the start position. In one motion, jump up and reverse your feet and arm positions. Perform thirty repetitions left and right on your first set, forty on your second.

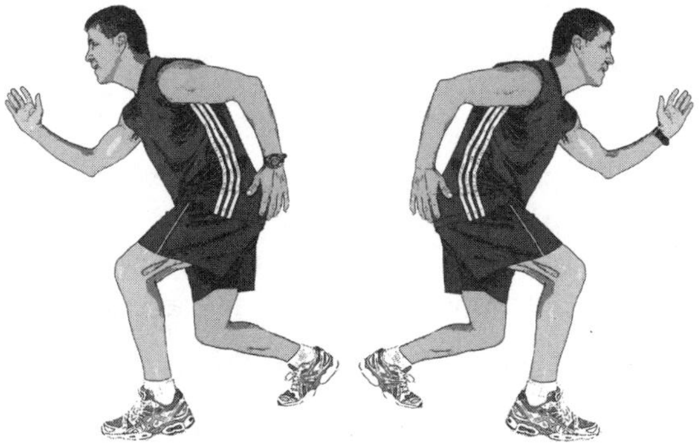

FIGURE 13.15 SPLIT JUMPS

Pointers

This exercise stretches your back and shoulders while strengthening your hips and core. Start by bending over and putting your right hand on the bench seat and putting all of your body weight on the ball of your left foot. Now, with your head down, extend your right leg and left arm at the same time, making your body into a parallel line with the floor; then switch to the opposite arm and leg. For the first set, perform fifteen repetitions on the right side and fifteen on the left. Perform twenty repetitions on each side for the second set.

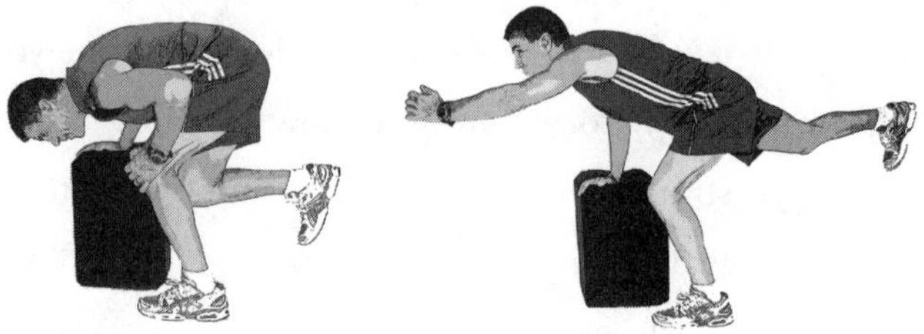

FIGURE 13.16 POINTERS

Four-Count Squat Thrusts

Another great whole-body exercise for the chest, shoulders, arms, and core is the four-count squat thrust. Assume a hip-width foot position with your hands on your hips. Count one, squat down and place your hands in a pushup position with arms extended. Count two, kick your legs straight back out, putting yourself in the complete upright pushup position. Count three, bring your feet back to your hands in a squat position. Count four, stand back up with your hands on your hips. Perform fifteen, four-count squat thrusts on your first set, and twenty on your second.

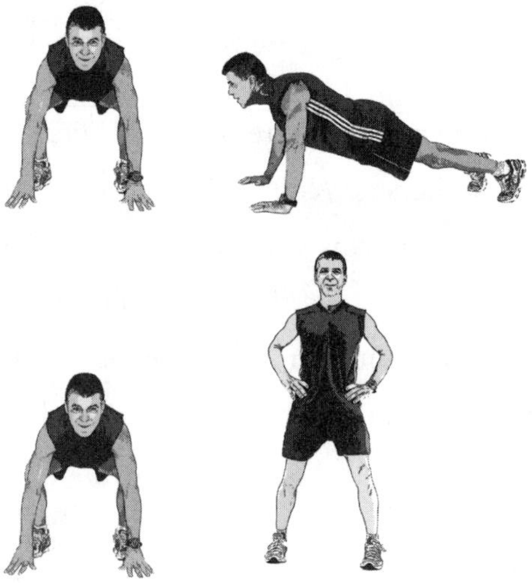

FIGURE 13.17 FOUR-COUNT SQUAT THRUSTS

Sky Reaches

This is an old-school, waist-reducing exercise that also strengthens your lower back. Assume the starting position with your hands on your hips. While keeping your head up and back slightly arched, squat down and place your fingertips on the ground between your feet. Stand back upright and reach your arms overhead while you slightly extend your back. Make sure to keep a bend in your knees. Perform twenty repetitions on the first set, twenty-five on the second.

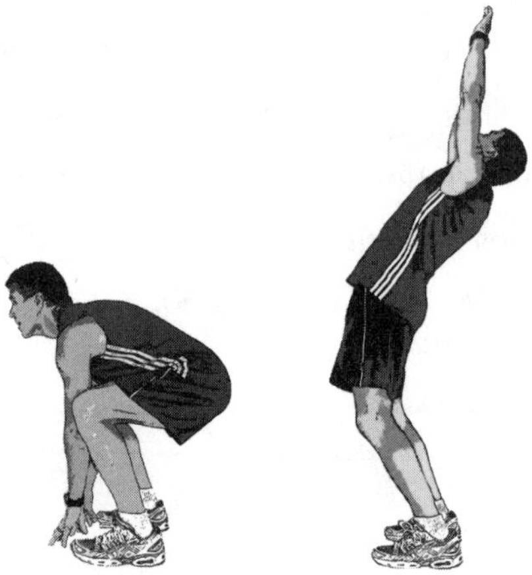

FIGURE 13.18 SKY REACHES

Well, I hope you enjoyed your workout. Although you are to go from exercise to exercise, I want you to always catch your breath. The inherent intensity of most of these eighteen exercises makes this workout predominantly anaerobic, and not aerobic. This type of training is the key to remaining young, supple, playful, and looking like a kid. I encourage you to do this workout with family and friends.

The Static Stretch Routine

Now I want to give you a stationary stretch routine that you can perform without having to go to the ground. I've been using this workout for over twenty-five years—I think you'll like it. You can perform these stretches at the end of your workouts to increase your range of motion, or you can use this routine to decompress, cool down, and relax.

Active Static Stretching

If you choose to strengthen your muscles as you hold these various stretches, you can apply moderate to maximum force while holding each stretch from twenty to, ideally, thirty seconds. If necessary, go ahead and perform as many sets of each stretch as you feel you need to gain improvement. Listen to your body and be careful not to overly force a movement.

Passive Static Stretching

If you want to bring the systems of your body down, perform these stretches more gently with light pressure. Make sure to breathe in a relaxed manner for both your mind and your body. Many of these stationary stretches have been done with added movement in your strength workout. This is a good thing because it makes you familiar with them and it gives continuity in your brain-body connection.

Sky Reaches

This is great for your shoulders, back, and rib cage. Assume a hip-width foot position with a slight bend in your knees. Extend your arms overhead and reach as high as you can. Hold the stretch for twenty to thirty seconds. Repeat if necessary.

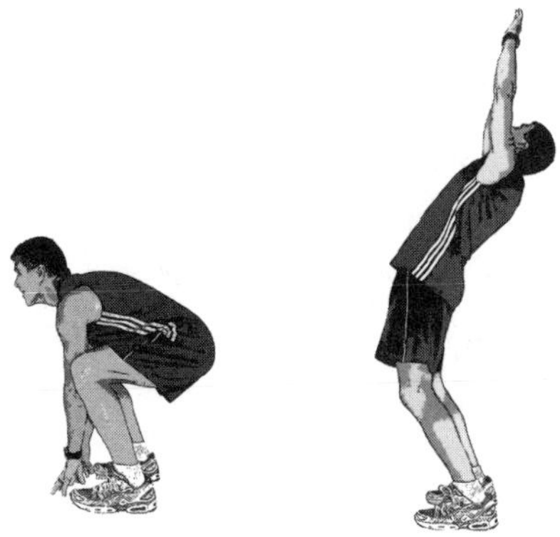

FIGURE 13.19 SKY REACHES

Pull-down Squeeze

Assume starting position. Reach to the sky with both arms, then pull your elbows straight down and back. Try to pinch your shoulder blades together. This is great stretch for your upper chest and your shoulders. All of your stretches should be held for twenty to thirty seconds.

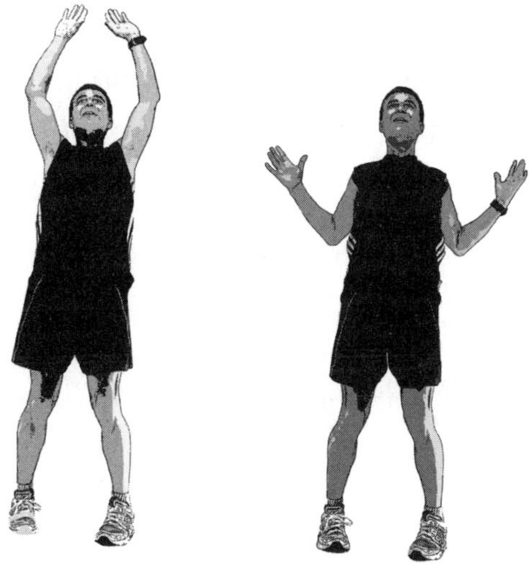

FIGURE 13.20 PULL-DOWN SQUEEZE

Cat Back

This is a great stretch for the rear shoulders and the entire upper back. Assume a hip-width foot position. Bring your hands together and extend your arms out in front. Round your middle back like a cat.

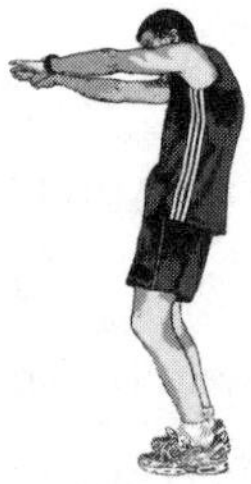

FIGURE 13.21 CAT BACK

Thumbs-up Row

This is a great posture exercise for your shoulders and upper back. Assume starting position. Extend your arms out in front. Now, pull your elbows straight back and together as you turn your thumbs up. Hold, applying moderate force for thirty seconds.

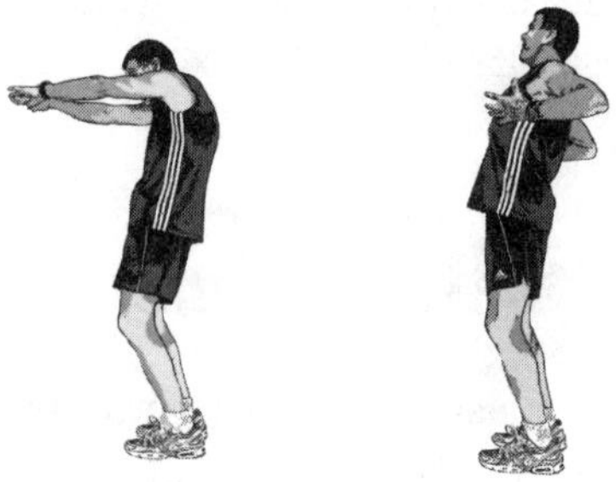

FIGURE 13.22 THUMBS-UP ROW

Hug Yourself

This is a two-part stretch for your outer upper back and side shoulders. Assume a hip-width foot position. Place your right arm over your left arm and hug yourself. Grip your shoulders with your hands. Hold this position for thirty seconds, and then switch arm positions.

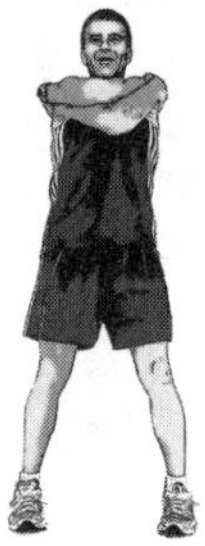

FIGURE 13.23 HUG YOURSELF

Cliff Diver

Assume a starting position with your knees slightly bent. With your elbows bent, pull your arms out and back while you arch your back. This is a great stretch for your chest.

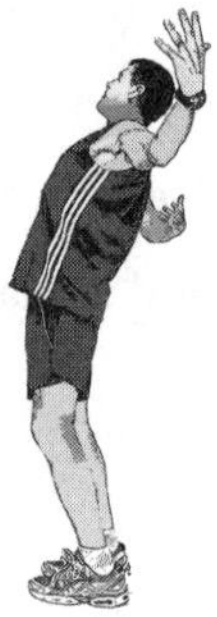

FIGURE 13.24 CLIFF DIVER

Rotary Twist

Assume a hip-width foot position. Bring your arms up in front of you at chest height. Rotate your upper body, looking as far to your left as possible. Hold for thirty seconds, and then rotate to your right.

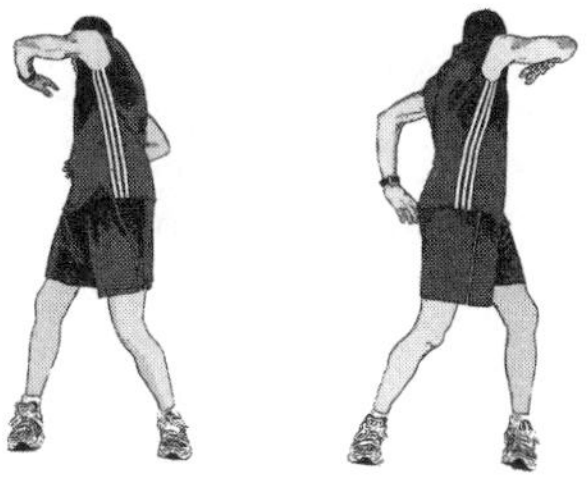

FIGURE 13.25 ROTARY TWIST

Side Bend

Assume a hip-width foot position. Put your left hand on your left thigh. Now, reach overhead with your right arm as you bend over laterally to your left. Hold this stretch for thirty seconds and then stretch to your right. This stretch is great for your shoulders, ribs, abdominals, and lower back.

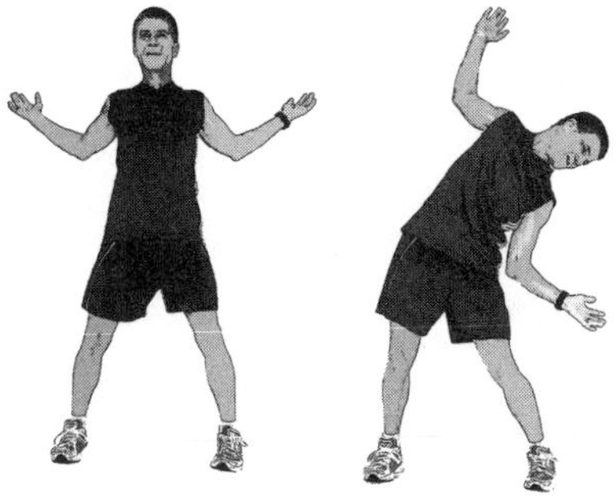

FIGURE 13.26 SIDE BEND

Full Squat

Assume starting position. Turn your toes slightly to the outside. With your head up and your lower back slightly arched, squat straight down, keeping your heels down. Extend your arms inside your knees and down in front of you. Relax your breathing and hold this stretch for the full thirty seconds. This is the best lower back and hip stretch, period!

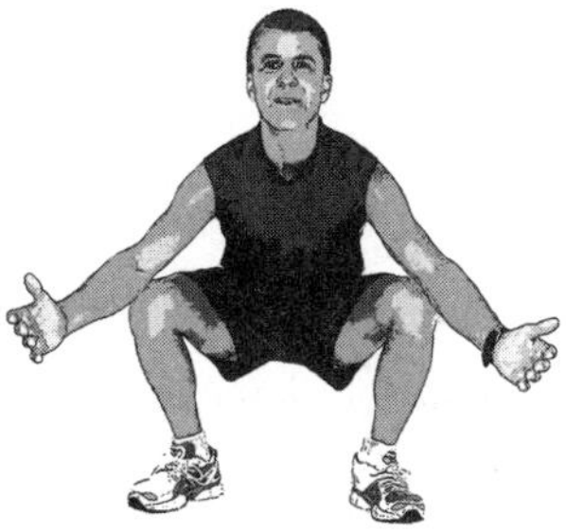

FIGURE 13.27 FULL SQUAT

Quad/Hip

If you can, try to stand and balance your body weight on your left foot. Reach down and grasp your right ankle. Pull your ankle and leg straight back, up, and out, stretching both your quad (front thigh) and front hip. Switch to the other side.

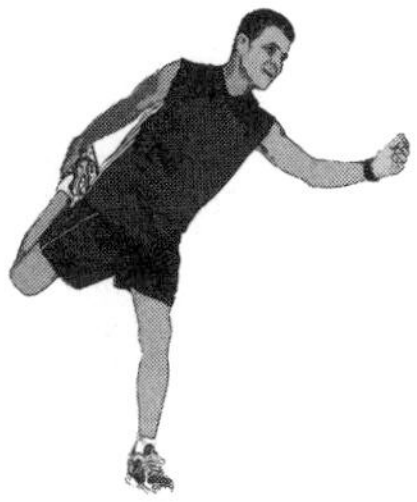

FIGURE 13.28 QUAD/HIP

Achilles/Calf

Assume a hip-width foot position and turn your toes straight forward. Now take a big step forward with your left leg. Put both hands on the top of your left thigh. While keeping your right heel flat on the ground, lean gently forward. Hold for thirty seconds and then switch foot positions. This is a great stretch for your calves, Achilles tendons, and the lower hamstrings.

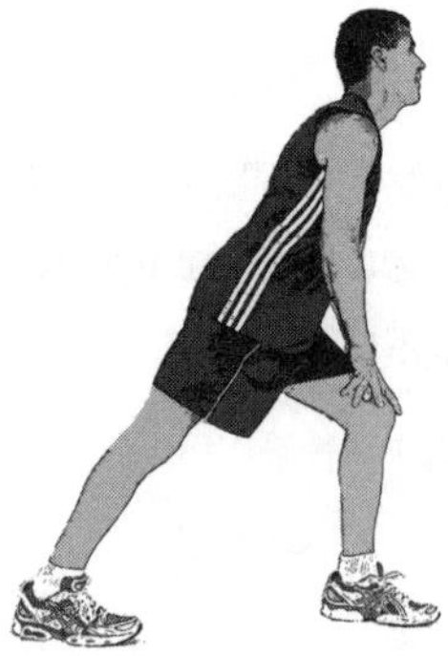

FIGURE 13.29 ACHILLES/CALF

Calf/Hamstring

Assume a hip-width foot position. Turn your left foot forty-five degrees to the outside. Now extend your right leg straight out in front of you with your heel on the ground. Flex your right toes back toward your knees, keeping your heel planted, and squat down until you feel a good stretch on your calf and hamstring. Hold for thirty seconds and switch leg positions.

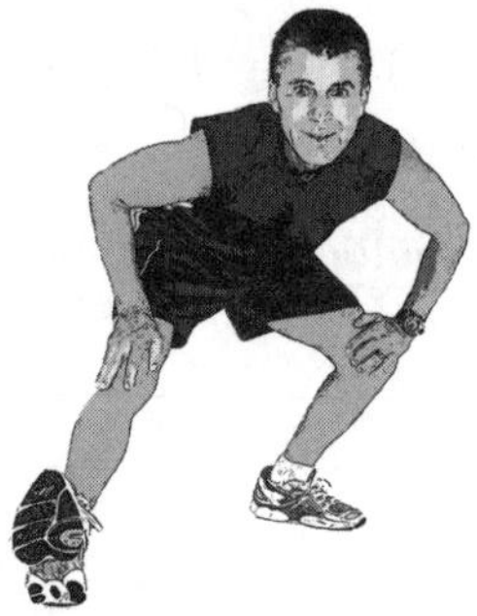

FIGURE 13.30 CALF/HAMSTRING

Calf/Groin

Assume a foot position much wider than hip-width. Put your hands on your right thigh as you slide laterally to your right. Fully straighten your left leg and sit into a squat, stretching your left groin and inside calf. Hold for thirty seconds, and then slide over to your left.

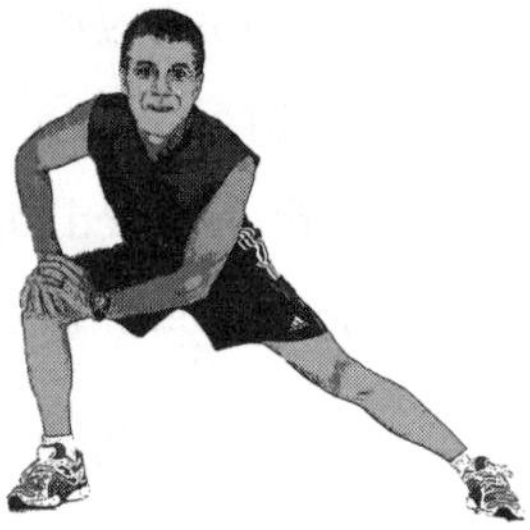

FIGURE 13.31 CALF/GROIN

Be Playful like a Kid

One of the keys to improving your flexibility and elasticity is to bend, twist, squat, and contort your body like a child does at a playground. By moving our bodies in these ways, we cause the hard, connective tissues to absorb body fluids and reach optimum volume. Water, the universal lubricant, is what gives your body its suppleness and pliability. The moment we stop moving our body and joints through their complete ranges of motion, they begin dehydrating and demineralizing. As our connective tissues dry up, they become rigid and inflexible. This brittleness leads to increased risk of injury and a much lower quality of life. So act like a kid, have fun, and be playful whenever possible. Playgrounds are for adults, too.

tip: Eat and Move

Work those lower abdominals with a set of lying flat leg raises. Sit down on the ground with your legs extended out in front of you. Now lay back so that you are propped up on your elbows and your hands are palm down flat. Point your toes and put a slight bend in your knees as you begin to do a set of fifteen leg raises. Raise your legs about a foot off the ground and then lower them gently back down.

Part Four: **Wrapping Things Up**

Participating in biblical physical fitness is one of the great keys to getting strong and overcoming stress and anxiety. It's not just because it ramps up your metabolic rate and burns off the deleterious effects of distress. Most important, it provides you with energy and electricity to fulfill God's will in and through your life.

DON'T WORRY, BE HAPPY, AND HAVE JOY

14

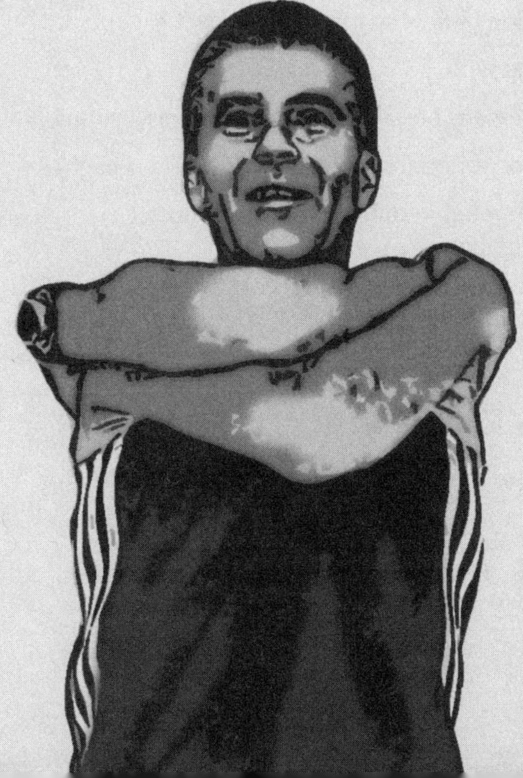

Back in the mid 1980s, I was part of a team of instructors that was presenting a three-day Police Officer Survival Seminar throughout the United States and Canada. My part was to teach the officers how to control their stress in high-risk situations and how to manage the effects of stress over the course of their careers. One of my co-presenters was a police psychologist. He would open his presentation with this definition of stress: Stress is not being able to choke someone who so richly deserves it.

Of course, he always got a good laugh. All joking aside, his definition was in part true. When we allow frustration, anger, and other feelings of emotional distress to build up over time without expressing or relieving this internal pressure, bad things can happen. Often we end up expressing severe stress in disastrous ways. Then we have to live the rest of our lives with consequences such as knowing we have inflicted pain on others. I know you've probably heard many times that you should never let emotional distress build up without dealing with it head-on, before it damages everyone. You've also probably heard to pause and count to ten before behaving rashly. To be honest with you, I include myself in this reminder. When we allow pressure to build up to the point that we lash out and say or do things in anger, it's because we have been spiritually weak. We have procrastinated in confronting the issues in a timely manner. The Bible is clear when it tells us that if we have a problem with someone or something, we should, in love, confront the problem. Most of the time, when we do act in obedience to the Scriptures, things work out for the best, and people get blessed. It's when we are weak and selfish that things turn out badly.

Hans Selye was a famous psychologist who gave the best definition of stress: any stimulus that places an adaptive demand on the systems of the mind, body, and organism (my paraphrase). Notice that stress is not inherently bad. In fact, by this definition, stress can be very good and productive. Selye added that only when stress goes beyond the capability of a person to adapt to it does it become destructive. Stress is a cause of premature death in America. Have you ever heard the adage that too much of a good thing can kill you?

In 2 Timothy 1:7 Paul says the Creator God gave us a fearless spirit of power, love, self-discipline, and a sound mind. The apostle Paul encourages us to use our heads and think things out before acting. Is it using your sound mind if you work yourself to death, yell at your spouse, or quit your job in a moment of rage? Are you using your sound mind when you lie around on the couch eating packaged, dead food, never getting any exercise? Our God-given, sound mind says no.

The Lord wants you and me to live in the now, not in the past and not in the future. In *The Screwtape Letters,* C. S. Lewis says that Satan captures our souls by keeping us distracted from the present and focused on our past or looking toward the future. Jesus himself told us in Matthew 6:34, "Don't worry about tomorrow, for tomorrow will bring its own worries. Today's trouble is enough for today."

In my original outline for this chapter, I was going to share all of the different sources of stress. But in the end, the only real cause of distress in our lives is ourselves. It's when we allow ourselves to neglect the Word of God and take our eyes off Jesus that we get ourselves into worry and trouble.

We lose joy when we choose to embrace negative thoughts. We can be an optimist or a pessimist. We can be trusting or skeptical. We can be generous or greedy. We can be thankful or demanding. We can look at the glass of water as being half full or half empty. You get the picture. We choose how we look at things. In Romans 12:2 Paul says:

> Don't copy the behavior and customs of this world, but let God transform you into a new person by changing the way you think. Then you will know what God wants you to do, and you will know how good and pleasant and perfect his will really is.

You'll notice it says to let God *transform* us. It's our decision to let God change our attitudes, the way we think.

Remember, stress isn't inherently good or bad. What's the opposite of any level of stress? No stress, right? However, if you have no stress acting upon you, forcing you to overcome and adapt, you're dead. It's stress that provides you with the zest for life. It's the victories that we have over ourselves that are the sweetest. When our mettle is tested, then we know who we really are. The Lord has provided trials and tribulations to refine and perfect us to become like him. The apostle Paul was chained to a dungeon wall, singing psalms and spiritual hymns. He was experiencing joy despite his circumstances. King Solomon said joy wasn't about wealth or position, but about our outlook. I don't know anyone who doesn't have some problems to deal with.

One of the persons I learned the most from as a young man was the motivational speaker and author Earl Nightingale. He shows what people worry about most:

- Things that never happen, 40 percent.
- Things from our past that can't be changed, 30 percent.
- Needless worries about our health, 12 percent.
- Petty miscellaneous worries, 10 percent.
- Real, legitimate worries, 8 percent.

Think about it! Ninety-two percent of the things most people worry about, things that consume valuable time, cause painful stress, even mental anguish, and are absolutely unnecessary! Again the Lord's Word openly talks about entertaining unnecessary fears, wrestling with one's thoughts, dwelling in your past, and spending time on nonproductive and dangerous worry. Of the real, legitimate worries—Nightingale's 8 percent—there are two kinds. One, problems we can solve, and two, those beyond our ability to solve. Usually, most of our real problems are the ones we can solve. We must learn how to take personal responsibility for solving them.

"Ninety-two percent of the things most people worry about are absolutely unnecessary."

One of my good friends from the Big Island of Hawaii likes to say, "Never let them see you sweat" and "Don't sweat the small stuff." I've added this saying: "Make everything small stuff, because it's small to God."

Here are five things to consider:

1. Your personality type
   Are you easygoing or hard-driving?
   Do you have a positive mental attitude?
   Do you laugh and smile a lot?
2. Your social relationships (you are who you hang with)
   Your friends
   Your family
   Your work environment
3. The environment you live in
   Noise pollution from traffic, sirens, and horns
   Air pollution from factories, waste disposal plants, and sewers
   Urban sprawl and lack of personal space
4. Toxic food
   Packaged, dead food that is genetically modified
   Food loaded with the poisons of preservatives, additives, and color dyes
   Foods contaminated with pesticides, fertilizers and growth hormones
5. Lack of movement (stagnation leads to disease and death)
   You've got to eat and move.
   Present your body to the Lord as a holy, living sacrifice through hard work and consistent exercise, day in and day out, week after week, month after month, and year after year.

Let's look at the Great Commission Jesus gave in Matthew 28:18–20.

> I have been given complete authority in heaven and on earth. Therefore, go and make disciples of all the nations, baptizing them in the name of the Father and the Son and the Holy Spirit. Teach these new disciples to obey all the commands I have given you. And be sure of this: I am with you always, even to the end of the age.

I believe the greatest distress comes from settling for mediocrity in your life. Almighty God created you for a specific purpose. There is no one who can do what you were destined to do, the way you can do it. To have joy, you must fulfill your destiny, beginning right now! Decide now to become as physically fit as you can for the rest of your life. Because, in doing so, you are loving the Lord your God with all of your heart, soul, mind, and strength.

Your attitude determines your altitude!

>> *tip:* Eat and Move

Let's get back to your core by doing a set of side bends. Assume a starting stance. Now keep your head forward and bring your arms back with a ninety-degree bend in then. Bend vertically to your left, touching your elbow to your hip, and then go to your right. Perform forty repetitions.

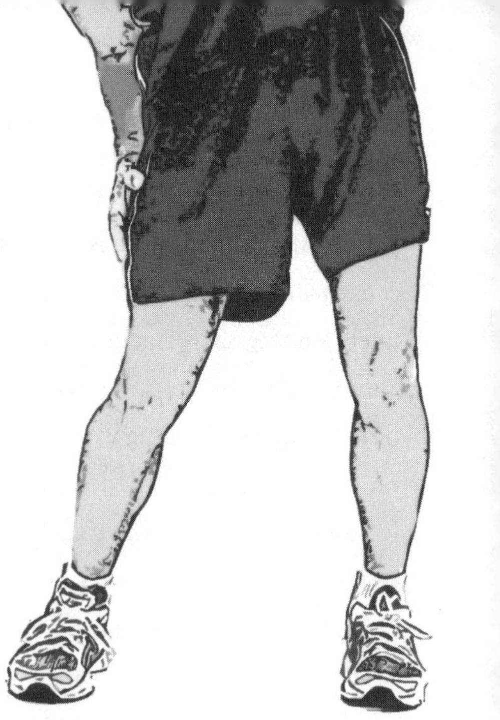

15

EXHORTATION AND A BLESSING

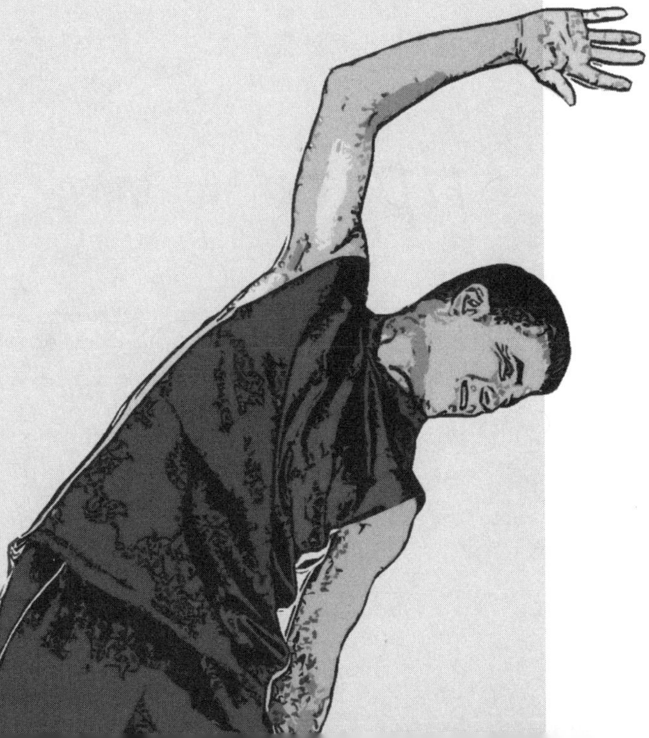

I wish you could feel the love and compassion that I have for you right now. I want you to know how proud I am of you for reading this book. I'm so thankful you have taken time to read and consider my experiences and beliefs. I leave you with the following exhortations.

Exhortations

- You can do this!
- You can become physically fit in your life. What one person can do, another can too. Have a fearless spirit.
- Awaken the sleeping giant within you!

  The Lord created you in his image and likeness. He made you a co-creator in the eternal scheme of things. The kingdom of God needs you to act and to offer the uniqueness and totality of your being for the good of humanity.
- Live day by day.

  Live now and fully experience every experience, every task that you have in front of you. Do it now!
- Make the grass deep green right where you are.

  You've been equipped with all the tools and equipment within your spirit and your soul to accomplish your mission.
- Make a commitment to excellence.

  The quality and joy of your life depend on your relentless and unwavering decision to always do your best.
- The only risk you have is in not taking any risk.

  If you want to walk on water, you have to get out of the boat. Where there is nothing to lose by trying and a great deal to gain by succeeding, try. And keep trying. Every adversity you face carries with it the seeds of even greater benefits.

- I dare you to aim high, because there is no one like you.

Hey, in heaven you're already famous.

The Blessing

The Lord created me, knew me, and determined my purpose before I was born. My consciousness of "I" began in 1957. Now, fifty years later, I am still discovering the mission he has set before me. My mission is to help you become physically fit according to the Scriptures. Rebecca and I believe the Holy Spirit gave us the name for this effort: Power and Might Ministries. In biblical terms, *power* and *might* mean *God's authority in action.* It's by this authority and this anointing that I pray this blessing over you:

> Father God, in the name of Jesus Christ—my Savior, my Brother, and my Master—I pray that those reading these words be infused and empowered by you to have a burning desire to become as physically fit as they can possibly become for the rest of their lives, and for your glory.
>
> I pray that you give them the strength and the courage to say yes to you and to the destiny that you have created them to achieve.
>
> I pray that they have the boldness, tenacity, and ferocity to say no to the devil and the powers of darkness who may come against them as they choose to become all they can be in "loving other humans as themselves."
>
> I pray that you will give them an excitement, an exhilaration, and a joy in the energies and electricity that are produced from a high level of physical fitness.
>
> Help them, Lord, to become acutely aware of the transformations that will occur within their mind, will, emotions, and physical body through their diligence and commitment to this lifelong journey.
>
> I pray health and longevity for their bodies and immortality for their spirits and souls in the kingdom of heaven.
>
> I pray that they will become their most perfect form in spirit, mind, and body, like the caterpillar that becomes a butterfly and the eaglet that becomes a majestic eagle.
>
> Lord, I pray your supernatural protection and anointing over my readers. You have predestined them to accomplish great things for you in their lives. Please, O Lord, give them this revelation. Do it, Lord! Please do it!
>
> As they finish reading this prayer of mine for them, overcome them with your Holy Spirit and shed light and love upon them.
>
> May their light shine brightly so everyone may see you, Lord, through their good deeds. And may their character, behavior, and lives be so salty that anyone who experiences them will want to know what they know and have what they have.
>
> May they be strong in you. Amen.
>
> Coach Powers
>
> In the year of our Lord, 2009

>> *tip:* Eat and Move

I know they're expensive, but have a half cup of fresh raspberries. I have to tell you that this is my favorite fruit. And to top it off, they have nutrient-dense seeds in them.

EPILOGUE: COACH'S STORY

16

Now that you've read this book through, you may be interested in my story. It's not necessary for you to read about my experiences, but I believe you'll feel my passion for physical fitness if you do. Also, seeing what motivates me may help you achieve your goals. I thought that it would be fun to structure my story in a timeline over the past fifty-four years. So here we go.

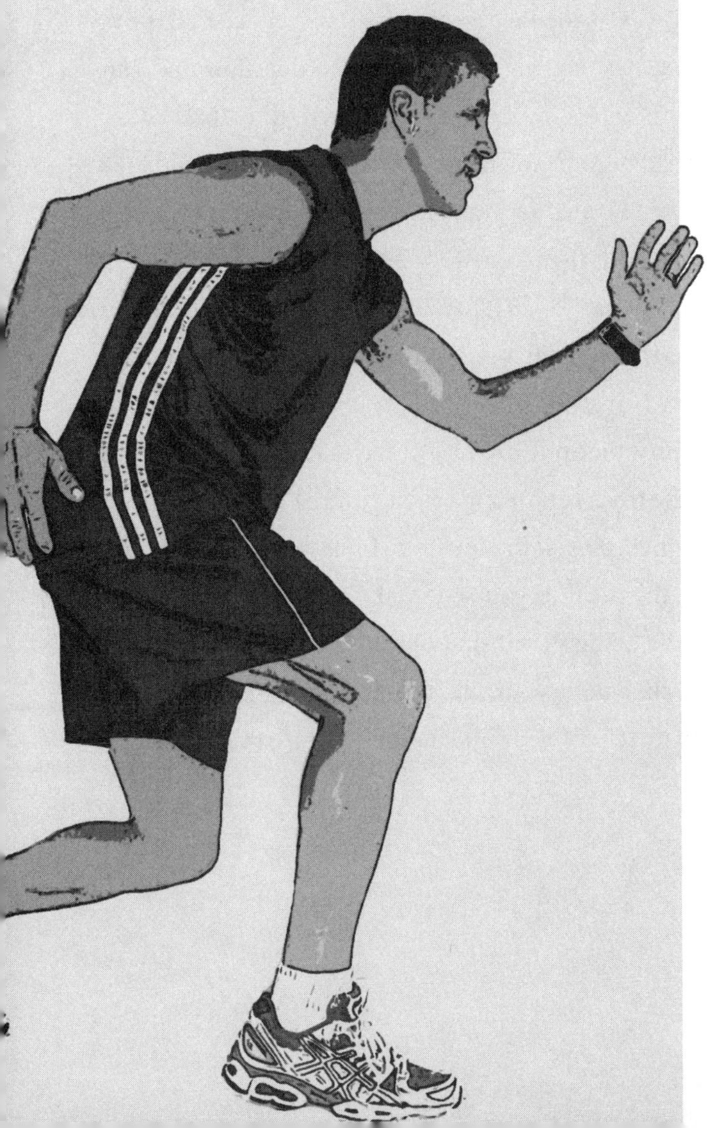

1957 Passionate Beginnings

I was born November 23, 1954, at Thanksgiving time. Approximately three years later, my Dad gave me my first memory. I can remember kneeling down on the living room floor next to him while he showed me how to do a pushups. Then he encouraged me to do as many as I could. Over the course of the next six years, he added additional calisthenics such as pull-ups and parallel dips. He even made me homemade, iron dumbbells and taught me how to perform bicep curls and shoulder raises. This was also when I learned how to box and wrestle, including the fun and competition of arm wrestling.

1963 Let's Get Physical

Third grade in Green Bay, Wisconsin, was a pivotal year. Even though I was overweight, I started participating in team sports. This was the Christmas I received my very first real set of barbells and dumbbells.

1965 The Olympic Lifts

At age eleven, my love of physical exercise went to another level. I started going to an evening weight-lifting program at our local community center. The coaches there taught me how to perform the official lifts for Olympic weight lifting.

1968 The Fitness Edge

By seventh grade, I was heavily involved in basketball and football. This was also the school year when I got rid of the fat. I finally figured out that you can't eat everything you want without your body becoming stuffed and plump. This was the year Dad told me, "A physically fit person has a distinct edge over people who aren't exercising regularly." I believed him then, and I believe him now.

1971 Sports Training Design

By 1971 I had been formally exercising and weight training for fourteen years. During my sophomore year of high school I began teaching other students, athletes, and even coaches what I'd learned about training with weights.

1974 I've Been Working on the Railroad

The most fun I ever had performing manual labor and the strongest I've ever been was the fall of 1974. I was working as a bridge and building carpenter for the Chicago and Northwest Railroad throughout northeastern Wisconsin. I also began undergraduate studies in criminal justice at the University of Wisconsin–Platteville. I absolutely loved this course of study and was fascinated by the teaching methodology. Although I could pick up the back end of an automobile, I weighed the heaviest I would ever become, 184 pounds.

1977 Oh, I Get It!

Although I had started watching what I ate in seventh grade, it wasn't until the winter of 1976–1977 that I came to realize my exercise and conditioning had to be balanced with eating nutritionally. This was also the time I started going to health and fitness clubs. The incredible array of exercise equipment and machines impressed me. I started studying exercise physiology and how and why humans move.

1979 Catastrophe and Despair

By the summer of 1979, I was running long distances, between 120 and 160 miles per week. My goal was to go to the Moscow Olympics on the U.S. marathon team. It may have been completely unrealistic, but it didn't matter because I was totally obsessed. My mother accused me of making running my god. There's no question that running was where my treasure was stored (Matt. 6:21). Running had become my identity. It was the way I could look the way I wanted to look and eat what I wanted to eat. I had a serious psychological disorder.

On August 15, 1979, I was out for my late afternoon, twelve-mile run. Ten miles into that run I felt a yank on my left hamstring. That yank was the first symptom of an injury that put me in a wheelchair temporarily and kept me from running for eight years. When I sat in front of the neurologist in Houston, Texas, he said, "Son, stop doing this stuff to yourself. Make a contribution to society. Stop being so selfish. Get a girlfriend. Do something productive with your life." I was forced to drop out of graduate school and come home to figure things out.

1980 Born Again

I began managing a number of fitness clubs in Chicago, Illinois, and northeast Wisconsin while I began rehabilitation for the nerves in my legs. By the spring of 1980, I could walk brief distances without an intense, burning pain in the back of my upper legs. There seemed to be some hope I was healing. I was still twenty pounds over my running weight, but I didn't really care about that anymore.

One evening, an extremely attractive young woman came into one of the health clubs inquiring about a membership. That was Rebecca, and she ultimately became my wife. Later that year, she shared the gospel of Jesus Christ with me. I accepted him as my Lord and Savior on October 11, 1980, at 10:15 in the morning.

1981 My Bride, My Partner

Rebecca and I were married June 5, 1981. That same year I became chief of police in a small town in Wisconsin. By the beginning of 1982, I was teaching police fitness at nearly all of the technical colleges throughout Wisconsin.

1983 One More Try

I was having a lot of fun as chief of police in that small town. I led parades, directed traffic, coached weight training for the high school, and counseled troubled youth. My wife and I were part of a community.

Although I still couldn't run without pain, my upper body was whole and injury-free. For whatever reason, I still had the bug to try and compete at an elite level in some endurance sport. I grew up paddling canoes on our lake and in Boy Scouts, so I contacted the U.S. Olympic canoeing coach. He said he was interested in giving me a tryout in Florida, so I went into training. Unfortunately, right before the junior nationals I injured a bursa sac in my right shoulder and back. That was that.

1985 Tactical Aerobics

By the summer of 1985, I had retired from police work. I devoted all of my efforts to my wife and two daughters, Michelle and Krista. By this time, I was a certified health and fitness instructor with the American College of Sports Medicine. I began traveling and speaking, presenting police training in physical fitness and defensive arrest tactics on a national level.

1987 I Can Run Again!

In the summer of 1987, eight years after my hamstring nerve injury, I could finally run long distances again, pain free. Praise God, I was healed!

During this time I founded the Fitness Institute for Police, Fire, and Rescue. I was also teaching instructors in seminars for national-level organizations and private corporations, such as the Justice System Training Association, Armament Systems and Procedures, and Calibre Press.

1991 Top of My Game

The winter of 1990–1991 proved to be the pinnacle of my career teaching fitness and use of force for police departments. I was now doing training seminars for police forces in Europe, Canada, Australia, and throughout the United States.

You can probably tell that my need to be famous and recognized was again crowding out my relationship with God. My insecurity and low self-esteem were driving me to self-promotion, criticism of my training colleagues, and weeks away from my wife and family. Although I had helped countless police officers survive the street and make the most of their careers, my motives were mostly selfish. By the end of 1994, my law enforcement and security service training career had bottomed out.

The year of 1995 was a wilderness for me. Depression and desperation are tremendous motivators. I was financially in debt and in need of everything, especially a clear voice from the Lord. His voice came that summer. "Are you done trying to *be* something?" He went on to tell me that I was already everything he had created me to be for his service.

1996 I Can See Clearly Now

During the summer of 1995, my family moved to East Texas. What wonderful people and a wonderful place to live. Within six months, the Lord whispered to me that I had left the primary medium he had destined for me to use to share his message—physical fitness. Now, restored in my joy, I had a clear path and a vision quest. Pure physical fitness had always been my favorite pastime. I began working as a fitness specialist for a very large health system in Tyler, Texas. Not long after that I received my professional certifications from the National Strength and Conditioning Association and the United States of America Weightlifting Federation.

By 1997 I had the great fortune of training primarily athletes. Soon into 1998, I founded the Texas Speed, Agility, and Quickness Academy. It became the sports science arm of the health system that I worked for.

1999 Standing before Kings

I had always heard that if you learned "a lot about a little" you would become an expert. By the fall of 1999, the Lord had made me a nationally recognized sport speed development expert. The fame was no longer about me; it was about directing others toward God through Jesus. From this time into 2002, he had me training U.S. Navy SEALs on the East and West coasts, NASCAR pit crew teams, and various professional athletes from Major League Baseball, the National Football League, and professional rodeo. It was so fun, and I'm so grateful to him for the opportunity.

2002 A New Adventure

By the spring of 2002, both Rebecca and I felt that the Lord wanted us to become directly involved with a worldwide ministry called Youth With A Mission (YWAM). We had received reports that there was an effort to begin an international evangelistic sports training program at YWAM's University of the Nations in Kailua-Kona, Hawaii. So, without any confusion or doubt, we sold everything we owned, mailed eight small boxes, and moved to the Big Island.

Over the course of the next five years, I worked as a professional trainer at local fitness facilities on the Kona coast. In the summer of 2003, I became the fitness director for a 3,200-acre, four-star resort. I held that position for three years before the Lord spoke to Rebecca and me again. This time, it was to go into full-time ministry.

2007 Physical Fitness Jubilee

In March of 2007, my wife and I launched Power and Might Ministries, Incorporated. The ministry has three components:

1. Presentations in churches of every denomination, explaining the divine concept of physical fitness in obedience to the Scriptures.
2. Two-hour "Fit to Serve" seminars for churches and Christian organizations, giving the components of physical fitness.
3. A Helps Ministry where Rebecca and I work directly, one-on-one, with church pastors, leaders, and missionaries, helping them get their bodies back in order.

Also, most recently, I established Vital Force International, a worldwide association of physical fitness instructors.

Well, this is it for now. I can't wait to see what the Lord has for us next. Let's all keep growing more into his image.

For information relating to Power and Might, Inc., presentations and seminars, please contact us at:

Website: www.powerandmight.org and

www.coachpowers.com

E-mail: coach@coachpowers.com

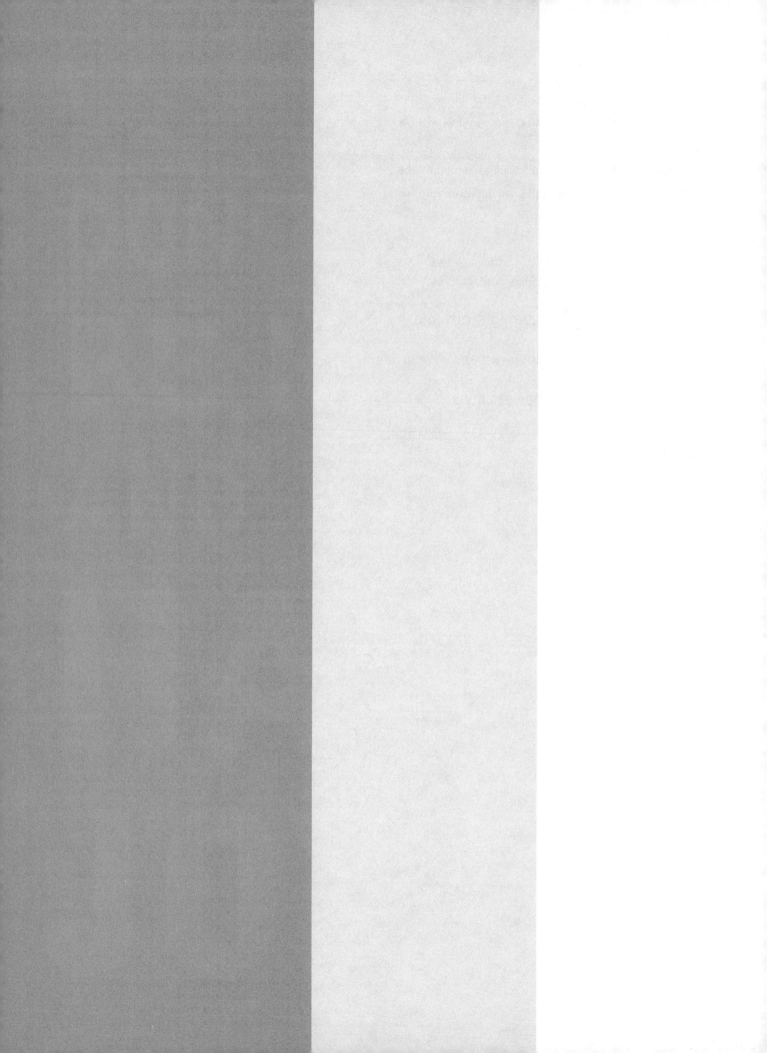

recommended reading

Colbert, Don. *The Seven Pillars of Health.* Lake Mary: Siloam, 2007.

Cunningham Siff, Mel. *Supertraining.* Denver: Supertraining Institute, 2003.

Morehouse, Laurence E., and Leonard Gross. *Maximum Performance.* New York: Simon & Schuster, 1977.

Ratey, John J. *A User's Guide to the Brain.* New York: Abacus, 2003.

Sears, Barry. *Enter the Zone.* New York: Regan Books, 1997.

The National Geographic Society Book Division. *Incredible Voyage: Exploring the Human Body.* Washington, D.C.: National Geographic Society, 1998.

gratitudes

Rather than just acknowledging those individuals who have helped me in the writing of this book, I want to give my heartfelt thanks and appreciation.

Of course, first, I want to thank the Godhead for creating the passion, joy, and excitement in my spirit, soul, and body for physical fitness and the continued pursuit of vitality.

Next, I want to thank my bride and wife of twenty-eight years, Rebecca, for her encouragement and ongoing support in the writing of this book and the overall ordaining of my destiny.

It was Loren Cunningham, the founder of Youth With A Mission (YWAM), who suggested, and almost insisted, that I write this book for the purposes of God and the benefit of others.

Special thanks go out to my editor, Jannie Cunningham-Rodgers, and her son, Jeff, for their help, trust, and support in this project.